Genetic databases

Over the past few years there has been a proliferation of genetic databases and biobanks, which promise to increase scientists' understandings of the way our genes interact with the environment. These biomedical research projects involve hundreds of thousands of people worldwide who are asked to donate blood and tissue samples as well as personal information. The control, exploitation and ownership of such detailed personal and medical information by governments and by commercial companies has generated social and ethical controversy.

Genetic databases offers a timely analysis of the underlying tensions, contradictions and limitations of the current regulatory frameworks for and policy debates about genetic databases. Drawing on original empirical research and theoretical debates in the fields of sociology, anthropology and legal studies, the contributors to this book challenge the prevailing orthodoxy of informed consent and explore the relationship between personal privacy and the public good. They also consider the multiple meanings attached to human tissue and the role of public consultations and commercial involvement in the creation and use of genetic databases.

The authors argue that policy and regulatory frameworks produce a representation of participation that is often at odds with the experiences and understandings of those taking part. The findings present a serious challenge for public policy to provide mechanisms to safeguard the welfare of individuals participating in genetic databases.

The book is written in an accessible style that will appeal to a multidisciplinary and international audience, and is relevant to policy discussions in Europe and in North America, as well as other countries that are developing similar initiatives. It will be of great interest to academics and students of medical sociology, health studies, public health, public policy and ethics.

Richard Tutton is a sociologist in the Science and Technology Studies Unit (SATSU) in the Department of Sociology at the University of York. His research has focused on the implications of genetic research and technologies for cultural identity and citizenship. **Oonagh Corrigan** is a sociologist with a research interest in social and ethical issues surrounding developments in genetics and the pharmaceutical industry. In particular, much of her work to date has focused on the implications for human subjects involved in biomedical research and on regulatory mechanisms designed to protect such subjects.

Genetic databases

Socio-ethical issues in the collection and use of DNA

Edited by Richard Tutton and Oonagh Corrigan

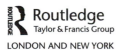
Routledge
Taylor & Francis Group

LONDON AND NEW YORK

First published 2004 by Routledge
11 New Fetter Lane, London EC4P 4EE

Simultaneously published in the USA and Canada
by Taylor & Francis Inc
29 West 35th Street, New York, NY 10001

Routledge is an imprint of the Taylor & Francis Group

Typeset in Garamond by Keystroke, Jacaranda Lodge, Wolverhampton
Printed and bound in Great Britain by TJ International Ltd, Padstow, Cornwall

Every effort has been made to ensure that the advice and information
in this book is true and accurate at the time of going to press. However,
neither the publisher nor the authors can accept any legal responsibility
or liability for any errors or omissions that may be made. In the case of
drug administration, any medical procedure or the use of technical
equipment mentioned within this book, you are strongly advised to
consult the manufacturer's guidelines.

British Library Cataloguing in Publication Data
A catalogue record for this book is available from the British Library

Library of Congress Cataloging in Publication Data
A catalog record for this book has been requested

ISBN 0–415–31679–0 (hbk)
ISBN 0–415–31680–4 (pbk)

Contents

Foreword

It is an honour and a pleasure to write the forward to this timely and exciting book, not only because this tightly-edited collection raises a specific set of issues about genetic databases, or addresses these so substantively, but because the collection sets an important benchmark for social scientific contributions to this field.

The rapid expansion of what might be called the social science of genomics poses a number of challenges. These are methodological, ethical, and political as well as being conceptual, empirical, and analytical. As this collection shows, the social science of genomics is profoundly interdisciplinary, not only combining many traditional areas of social science, from anthropology to economics, but also moving across into the clinical and scientific disciplines. While the social science of genomics will draw on science studies, cultural studies, and gender studies, it will also turn back to some of the oldest conceptual traditions in the social sciences, such as the debates about gift exchange, the formation of capital, or the meaning of reproductive substance.

There are a number of risks for the field due to the speed of expansion of genomics studies areas, the influx of large numbers of new researchers into the field, and the pressure on researchers to respond to so many varied constituencies – from granting bodies to policy and regulatory planners, as well as the government and industry. These are pressures the contributors to this book handle with both diligence and clarity. It is inspiring and refreshing to see the very high level of critical scholarly analysis that is maintained throughout the volume.

This is largely due to the skill and hard work of each of the contributors. But it is also the result of the foresight of the editors, Richard Tutton and Oonagh Corrigan, who have identified such an important topic, and brought together the contributors who could produce such a superb anthology. What we have as a result is a model of what we might hope to see for this field as a whole in a few years time. What this book offers that is perhaps its greatest achievement is the possibility of a comparative view. By bringing together contributors from a range of different countries, each of whom is addressing a different aspect of genetic databases, we are able both to read each specific chapter or case, and then reconsider them against other cases and perspectives.

What is equally important is the level of empirical detail provided by the contributors, for these perspectives will tell us what happens 'when the rubber meets the road', which may be a far cry from what was promised, intended, or imagined. For example, while it is widely acknowledged that the principle of informed consent is problematic in the context of genetic donation, we will need to know much more about why and how this is so before we will be able to propose practical ethical alternatives. Without the kind of detailed studies of the actual relations and practices that shape the conditions of genetic donation, we will not have enough information to produce an informed critical account of them. And ultimately, such an account will work best when it can be comparative, which, again, is what is so important about this volume. It sets an inspiring example for the future of the social science of genomics, and it is a credit to all of those whose contributions have made it possible.

Professor Sarah Franklin, Lancaster University, December 2003

Contributors

Richard Ashcroft Primary Health Care and Medicine, Imperial College, 324 Reynolds Building, Charing Cross Campus, St Dunstan's Road, London W6 8RP, UK

Helen Busby IGBIS, University of Nottingham, Law and Social Sciences Building, University Park, Nottingham NG7 2RD, UK

Oonagh Corrigan Centre for Family Research, Department of SPS, University of Cambridge, Free School Lane, Cambridge CB2 3RF, UK

Trudy Goodenough University of Bristol, Centre for Ethics in Medicine, 73 St. Michael's Hill, Bristol BS2 8BH, UK

Erica Haimes Department of Sociology and Social Policy, University of Newcastle, Newcastle upon Tyne NE1 7RU, UK

Klaus Hoeyer Institute of Public Health, University of Copenhagen, Blegdamsveg, DK 2200, Copenhagen N, Denmark

Jane Kaye ETHOX, Institute of Health Sciences, University of Oxford, Oxford OX3 7LF, UK

Julie Kent Faculty of Humanities, Languages and Social Sciences, University of the West of England, Coldharbour Lane, Bristol BS16 1QY, UK

Graham Lewis SATSU, Department of Sociology, University of York, York YO10 5DD, UK

Richard Tutton SATSU, Department of Sociology, University of York, York YO10 5DD, UK

Sue Weldon Centre for the Study of Environmental Change, Institute for Environment, Philosophy and Public Policy, Furness College, Lancaster University, Lancaster LA1 4YG, UK

Michael Whong-Barr Department of Sociology and Social Policy, University of Newcastle, Newcastle upon Tyne NE1 7RU, UK

Emma Williamson University of Bristol, Centre for Ethics in Medicine, 73 St. Michael's Hill, Bristol BS2 8BH, UK

Acknowledgements

A number of people have helped us in the editing of this book and we would like to thank Anne Kerr, Sarah Cunningham-Burley, Martin Richards, Andrew Webster, Sarah Franklin, Nik Brown and Graham Lewis for providing valuable advice, insights and comments at various stages in the life of this project. We would also like to thank the contributors for their hard work, whose quality of research and writing made the editing process an enjoyable and stimulating one. We dedicate this book to D, Ben and Hannah.

Richard Tutton and Oonagh Corrigan, The Editors

Chapter I

Introduction

Public participation in genetic databases

Richard Tutton and Oonagh Corrigan

Even before the celebratory announcement in June 2000 that 90 per cent of the human genome sequence had been completed, it seems that the post-genomic era was already taking shape. In Iceland, Britain, Estonia and elsewhere plans were being put in place for the creation of genetic databases, presented by their advocates as the next progressive step forward from the Human Genome Project. These databases are distinctive by the way that they combine genetic information derived from blood samples with various kinds of personal data about medical history, lifestyle or genealogy from thousands or hundreds of thousands of ordinary people across national or regional territories. They are potentially the key to developing scientific understanding of and therapeutic treatments for common multifactorial diseases, as well as determining why groups of people have differing reactions to pharmaceutical drugs.

The creation of genetic databases has been surrounded by controversy and debate, attracting worldwide media attention and significant financial investment by both public and private bodies. At national and international levels, policy-makers have sought to define and engage with what they see as the considerable social, ethical and legal issues at stake.[1] These include informed consent, commercialization, ownership, privacy, confidentiality and public confidence in the governance of research. Many of these are long-standing areas of public policy in relation to the new genetics more broadly, but genetic databases raise specific and sometimes novel questions in relation to these areas, with the result that many have become the subject of renewed policy debate. The chapters in this book should be seen in this context. They present a significant contribution to an understanding of the social and ethical aspects of the ways people come to participate in genetic databases, both as donors of tissue samples and personal information and as participants in public consultations on the formation and governance of these projects. In different ways, the starting point for the chapters is a critique of the regulatory frameworks or social representations that have emerged from policy discourses related to genetic databases. Some chapters present the findings of much-needed empirical research on the perspectives of research participants in different genetic database projects; others focus their analysis on the history and language of policy discourses themselves. The exception to this is Graham Lewis' chapter that provides an overdue account of the increasingly significant but under-reported commercial context of tissue collection and genetic databases. Written in an accessible style by researchers with backgrounds in sociology, science studies, anthropology and law, the book addresses the multi-dimensionality of the issues at stake in genetic databases for a multidisciplinary and international audience. It contributes both to a developing body of academic research and is highly relevant for public policy.

There has been some debate about what is meant by a genetic database, how they differ from earlier forms of databases (Chadwick and Berg 2001), and which of the various terms – genetic database, biobank, DNA bank, genetic databank, population database or population collection – is the most appropriate to use.[2] The question of definition is one with implications for policy-making and the direction of academic research. When the UK House of Lords Science and Technology Committee issued its report on 'human genetic databases' it used this term to describe 'collections of genetic sequence information, or of human tissue from which such information might be derived, that are or could be linked to named individuals' (House of Lords 2001). While appearing to be very broad, this definition deliberately excludes personal, medical or genealogical data. In written evidence to this committee, Paul Martin (2000) argued that genetic databases involved the integration of genotype data (as derived from tissue samples) and medical data. This is an essential feature of these kinds of projects since the research on gene association or 'gene–environment' interactions depends precisely on the interplay of these different datasets. Martin concluded that policy discussions in relation to genetic databases therefore have to deal with issues arising from both the use of personal and genetic information, which may otherwise be seen as separate concerns. As Ruth Chadwick and Kare Berg (2001) note, some of the 'most complex ethical issues arise when [DNA samples] are linked to health records' (Chadwick and Berg 2001: 318). While narrow in one respect the House of Lords' position is of interest in that it implies genetic databases are assemblages of what Bronwyn Parry (2003, 2004) calls the 'corporeal' and the 'informa-tional', holding both physical tissue and electronic data. However, for some this is just 'muddying the waters', and they would prefer a clear separation made between collections of tissue and the databases of information associated with them (King 2000).

Mention should also be made of the term 'biobank' that has particular prevalence in Scandinavia and increasingly so in Britain through the UK Biobank initiative (which we discuss below). When introducing the findings of a research project undertaken in Sweden on human biobanks, Mats Hansson (2001) suggests that, as a working definition, they can be understood as 'collections of human biological material within the health care system and the medical sciences' (Hansson 2001: v). This emphasis on the biological over the informational is borne out in many of the papers produced by the project's researchers, which focus on aspects of the provision of tissue samples rather than that of different kinds of personal data. However, others do highlight the relationship between genetic and clinical information as a key feature of biobanks (see Laage-Hellman 2001). In Britain it is unclear how the term has come to be used. However, one may observe that the name UK Biobank does distance this project from the National DNA Database used by the forensic science service in matters of criminal investigation (Guillén *et al.* 2002).

At best, there is some ambiguity surrounding these projects in which significant scientific and commercial investment is being made. For ease, we use the term genetic database in this introduction. However, some of the contributors to this book prefer to use other terms and we have not sought as editors to impose a uniform nomenclature. Most important is an understanding of what constitutes a genetic database or a biobank: as we made clear in the opening paragraph, we depart from the position of the House of Lords in that we see these databases as involving the collection, storage and use of physical tissue (usually blood, but by no means exclusively so), genotype and other biological information derived from that tissue, and a variety of personal data from populations of various sizes.

Moreover, these people tend to be healthy, which is to say they are not patients undergoing treatment. This is a significant difference from earlier and ongoing disease registries and databases, which we do not look at in this book.[3] The exception to this are those participants in clinical trials who are increasingly being asked by researchers on behalf of pharmaceutical companies to provide tissue samples. Many of these are indeed patients suffering from various conditions. But on the whole genetic databases are distinctive in enrolling large numbers of people who are currently not unwell. We do concur with the House of Lords in viewing genetic databases as combining both the 'corporeal' and the 'informational', the interplay of which raises certain ethical, legal and social issues discussed by some of the contributors here. Most of the genetic databases discussed in this book share these characteristics despite the different ways in which they are described either by the institutions behind them or by authors in their chapters.

The ambiguity about definition, which, as we have suggested, has direct relevance for policy-making and academic commentary, is part of a wider confusion that seems to surround many genetic database projects. The inception and development of genetic databases are fluid and sometimes not very transparent processes with numerous actors involved, many of whom may have scientific or commercial interests to protect. In the most controversial of cases, these projects are also enveloped by the claims and counter-claims of their supporters and opponents. All this makes any full account of these projects difficult. Indeed, the writing of a comprehensive scientific and social history of genetic databases will be a challenging task and is not one that we attempt here. However, to preface a discussion of the chapters in this book, we outline some of the particular developments that have come to dominate our view of genetic databases.

Charting the rise of genetic databases

Academic, policy and journalistic commentary on the global phenomenon of genetic databases has tended to centre on a number of high profile projects that have appeared since 1997. The first and probably most controversial is the Icelandic Biogenetic Project, which is being developed by a commercial company, deCODE Genetics, licensed by the Icelandic Government to construct and operate various public and proprietary databases under this rubric (Pálsson 2002).[4] The database that has attracted most attention is the proposed Health Sector Database. Contentiously, the organizers departed from the norm of informed consent, requiring individuals to 'opt-out' to avoid inclusion of their data (Kaye and Martin 2000). The stated purpose of this database is to assist the identification of genes involved in common diseases, such as diabetes (deCODE Genetics 2003).

Inspired by the Icelandic project, but also learning from the controversy that surrounded it, two further proposals for large genetic databases followed in Britain and Estonia. In 1998, the UK Medical Research Council (MRC) and the Wellcome Trust, Britain's largest medical research charity (joined later by the UK Government's Department of Health) combined forces to develop proposals for a genetic database (Hagmann 2000, McKie 2000a, 2000b, POST 2002, Barbour 2003). Rather than cover the entire population, this is a large-scale cohort of 500,000 people in the 45–69 age range. Originally called the UK Population Biomedical Collection, and now known as UK Biobank, beginning in 2003–04 it will start collecting blood samples, medical and lifestyle details from volunteers who will participate on a voluntary opt-in basis.[5] These volunteers will not have the right to receive personal feedback on the genetic information derived from their samples. UK Biobank will be run by a charitable, not-for-profit company and will be primarily an academic enterprise but with commercial access to and use of the database. The overall aim of UK Biobank is to study the interactions between people's genetic make-up, their experience of health and disease, as well as their lifestyles to determine the underlying epidemiological processes involved in the development of common diseases (UK Biobank 2003).

During the same period as these developments in Britain, an alliance of scientists in Estonia were involved in creating the Estonian Genome Foundation with the express purpose of creating a genetic database to hold blood samples, as well as personal data gathered from interviews with donors about their health, lifestyle and family history. This became known as the Estonian Genome Project. The development of this initiative took a legislative route as in Iceland and the Estonian Genome Project Foundation was formed to oversee its operation, which is accountable to the Department of Health in the Estonian government. Commercial exploitation of the database side is licensed to a spin-out company called EGeen, based in California (Estonian Genome Project 2003, Mieszkowski 2003). Notably, donors to the project do have the right to access the genetic information derived from their donated tissue sample. This is so they can gain from the anticipated benefits of pharma-cogenetics in the future (Estonian Genome Project 2003). As with UK Biobank, participation is on a voluntary opt-in basis with informed consent.

An initiative supported by the Tongan government to create a genetic database, which would have been licensed to an Australian biotechnology company, has also been noteworthy because by contrast it has so far been unsuccessful (Nowak 2000, Burton 2002). This database would have included health and genetic information to be used for research into common diseases, specifically diabetes and obesity, and people would have participated on a voluntary opt-in basis. It was also reported that the Tongan government and the company involved, Autogen, had reached a profit-sharing agreement (Nowak 2000). The idea for a national genetic database met with strong oppo-sition from church groups and those campaigning for transparent government in Tonga. The plans for the database were developed largely without public involvement and without consideration of the extended family networks that characterize Tongan society, which problematized the emphasis Autogen gave to individual informed consent (Burton 2002).

As well as these national projects, the formation of a database in the Canadian province of Newfoundland and Labrador has also attracted attention both in North America and Europe (Atkinson 2000, Meek 2000, Staples 2000). In 2000 a British biotechnology company, Gemini Holdings (that merged in 2001 with the US company Sequenom) struck an alliance with a consortium of Newfoundland-based researchers to set up Newfound Genomics, a commercial company, to operate a database of genetic and genealogical information collected from both the healthy population and from families who have diseases commonly found in the province. The database is being run on a voluntary opt-in basis with informed consent and aims to increase understanding of the role genes play in disease with the ultimate hope of producing new drug interventions. Other smaller-scale regional or local databases are in the process of being created, such as in Quebec (Staples 2000) and across the United States where the absence of a national healthcare system means that clinics are taking the lead in creating databases on the popula-tions in their specific areas (Kaiser 2002a). These have many of the same characteristics as the databases we have described so far.

Other, perhaps not so well known, national database projects are in the process of being set up in Latvia and Singapore. The Latvian Genome Project, created by legislation in 2001, is modelled closely on its counterpart in neigh-bouring Estonia (Abbott 2001). A pilot project was undertaken in 2001–03, leading to the planned establishment of the database itself over the following six years. The Latvian Genome Project is funded by the national government through its Council of Science and is part of its efforts to build national capacity in the areas of human genetic and biological sciences (Unified Genome Database of Latvian Population 2003). Another ongoing project is being undertaken in Singapore where a government body, the Singapore Genomics Programme, is developing a national database of medical, genealogical and genetic information. Initially this will be collected from patients with common diseases, but there are plans to include the entire population (Cyranoski 2000).

While much attention has been given to many of these new genetic databases in which national or regional public bodies have been involved to varying degrees in partnership with commercial companies, the pharmaceutical and genomics industries have been involved in creating their own proprietary databases (Martin 2001, Kaiser 2002a, 2002b). In this volume Graham Lewis and Oonagh Corrigan both address this aspect of the development of genetic databases, as we discuss below. There also exist databases that predate those so far discussed that have recently become the sites of commercial interest. As in the case of the Framingham Heart Study in Massachusetts, a database of genetic and health data run by the National Institutes of Health, this can be particularly controversial (Connolly 2000). There was strong public opposition to what was perceived to be profiteering from publicly owned resources, raising questions about what the economic return should be from the commercial exploitation of publicly funded research. Another example is the Medical Biobank in Västerbotten, northern Sweden that holds DNA and other biological samples as well as lifestyle and medical data on 66,000 people in the region. This biobank has been in existence since 1987 and is linked with several high-quality disease registers (UmanGenomics 2003). In 1999 a company, UmanGenomics, was created in order to realize the commercial potential of the biobank (UmanGenomics 2003). Klaus Hoeyer addresses issues of public participation in this biobank in chapter 6.

There also exist regional databases in Britain such as the North Cumbria Community Genetics Project (NCCGP) (Chase et al. 1997) and the Avon Longitudinal Study of Parents and Children (ALSPAC) (ALSPAC 2003) that date more than ten years in terms of their original conception. Both of these projects are birth cohort databases that collect a variety of tissue samples and personal information relating to health, lifestyle and family environment from both children and adults. Together they involve around 30,000 people. This book presents findings from important empirical sociological research on public participation in both the NCCGP and ALSPAC, respectively, by Erica Haimes and Michael Whong-Barr; and Emma Williamson, Trudy Goodenough, Julie Kent and Richard Ashcroft. The results of these studies will be highly relevant for the larger-scale database projects that have attracted much more public interest nationally and internationally.

The field of genetic databases is then a complex one, but the picture sketched here in the broadest of brush strokes provides the background to the research presented in this book, which examines the social and ethical aspects of public participation in these biomedical research projects. We introduce the chapters through three key themes of languages of participation, consent and control, and commercialization, but this should be seen as merely heuristic: the reader will find that almost all the chapters address these themes in one way or the other.

Languages of participation

Continuing the theme of language begun at the outset, one of the key concerns explored in this book is the way in which public participation in research is represented in policy discourses. There is no neutral language in which to talk about 'public participation' (a phrase which is itself problematic) in genetic databases. One encounters different ways of speaking about the provision or donation or giving or taking of human tissue and personal data, and about the people involved as sources or donors or participants. More specifically, one may find terms such as 'tissue donor' (Smaglik 2000) or 'gene donor' (Nature 1996, Estonian Genome Project 2003) used, and this impacts on an understanding of where value lies in relation to the material involved. Through these languages people are conceived as certain kinds of research subjects within fields of governmentality in relation to institutions. These languages are informed by assumptions about the nature of people's involvement with research, their motives for doing what they do, which draw on concepts from domains such as bioethics, philosophy, anthropology or law. Such language may be used by policy-makers to produce particular representations of research that serves scientific, commercial or political interests.

One such language is that of 'gift', used in the British context to conceptualize the provision of tissue by individuals to biomedical researchers. Such a language is influenced by Richard Titmuss' seminal account of blood donation in the UK during the 1960s and Richard Tutton's chapter reveals how this has been used in ethical discourses that oppose the continuing commodification of human tissue. Tutton examines how the language of gift and 'gift relationships' is deployed to envisage a model of public participation in biomedical research, through the provision of tissue samples, as altruistic and as resisting the commodification of the human body. It does so by creating a boundary between what can and cannot be commercialized that also determines who can and cannot financially benefit from the exploitation of tissue. His discussion is based primarily on two examples of recent ethical guidelines on the use of human tissue. The first was produced by the Nuffield Council on Bioethics in 1995, the other by the Medical Research Council in 2001. Both sets of guidelines are based on a model of biomedical research that involves some kind of public–private partnership. Tutton challenges the continuing use of the language of gift with respect to 'genetic donation' and suggests there is a need to adopt a different approach to the question of how human tissue provided for research should be conceived and regulated. He argues that we need a more transparent approach to the development of guidelines, which would take into account both the specificities of the tissue and the fact that its scientific and commercial value lies in the genetic information derived from it.

Helen Busby also engages with the languages of policy discourses, which draw on abstract theories from bioethics and law to produce accounts of voluntary participation in research. Her aim is to challenge these accounts and the assumptions underlying them, especially in terms of their key mobilizing concepts such as 'gift', informed consent and expertise. Busby argues that empirical research is needed in order to highlight and address the specific social and cultural dimensions of these concepts that tend to be overlooked by bioethicists. Her research involves two case studies, using one of blood donors to the UK National Blood Service as a reference point for examining participation in a genetic research project. Linking these studies both through the common biological substance donated as well as the influence that Tutton noted of Titmuss' work on 'gift relationships' – Busby discusses issues to do with trust and knowledge. She argues that contrary to the emphasis in bioethics on the importance of conveying greater levels of information as a way of facilitating trust, this arises as much from the perceptions of and relationships with institutions, such as the UK National Health Service or universities. Busby posits that people, who are often working at the limits of expertise in these contexts, are willing to 'entrust' what they have given to these kinds of institutions. Another key theme to emerge from Busby's chapter is that of reciprocity, which she finds very much in evidence amongst blood transfusion donors but which is lacking in current policy discussions about genetic databases such as UK Biobank. Busby concludes that public expectation of some form of reciprocity needs to be acknowledged and met if such initiatives are to gain public trust.

Erica Haimes and Michael Whong-Barr also challenge some of the underlying concepts in policy discourses around public participation by presenting findings from a study investigating the views, values and reasons for the agreement or refusal of women who, during pregnancy, have been asked to donate tissue samples and lifestyle data for the UK's North Cumbria Community Genetics Project. Drawing upon interviews with the research team and those women who both donated and refused, this chapter analyses the variations in the meanings and processes attached to the decision-making process. The authors challenge the categories 'agreement' and 'refusal' used to describe responses to the request to provide DNA samples and information showing that the distinction between 'donors' or 'non-donors' is rather more nuanced. Rather than use the terms 'donation' or 'non-donation', which imply a single meaning attached to a simple one-way act, they use the notion of 'participation' to begin to reflect what is in fact a highly varied social process with multiple meanings. They discuss the context in which the request to donate to such a database lies and the associated issues raised by the responses to this request, at both individual and community levels. They also examine the socially powerful discourse of altruism and find that non-participants feel a generalized cultural pressure or imperative to donate and to help, which is perhaps particularly acute during pregnancy when they are recipients of much medical help and support. The authors suggest that those who do participate are not necessarily as altruistic as is usually assumed and that those who do not participate are as equally altruistic as their participating counterparts. This chapter contributes much needed insight to inform the debates about how participation in genetic databases should be understood.

Consent and control

Probably the single most debated issue in relation to genetic databases is that of consent (Lyttle 1997, Beskow *et al.* 2001, Chadwick and Berg 2001, Caulfield 2002, Sade 2002, Caulfield *et al.* 2003). There is nothing particularly new about this issue as bioethicists and policy-makers have hotly discussed notions of consent for decades. In particular, informed consent in the context of biomedical research has been gaining increasing significance since it first appeared in international guidelines over fifty years ago (Corrigan 2003). But in the context of genetic databases a number of specific issues have arisen that has led to a renewed debate about the limits of current consent models and whether new, different notions of consent need to be considered. This relates not only to participation in operational databases but also to the processes by which new databases come into being.

Oonagh Corrigan's discussion traces the development of informed consent through a number of international ethical codes of practice, developed since the atrocities of Nazi doctors in the Second World War, as the solution to the potential dangers posed to individuals by their participation in medical research. She situates the emergence and establishment of informed consent within the broader contexts of Western moral philosophy and more recent human rights discourses. Drawing on the writings of Michel Foucault as well as more recent discussions about 'active citizenship' within sociology, she argues that the process of informed consent entails the construction of 'biological citizens', with a right to be informed about the research in which they may chose to participate and a responsibility to make those choices informed and rational ones. The substantive context of her chapter is that of clinical drug trials, which are becoming increasingly important sources of human tissue samples as patients and healthy volunteers are routinely asked to provide some of their tissue to be used for long-term pharmacogenetics research. Corrigan sees these trials as highlighting the inadequacies of the practice of informed consent. With the add-on pharmacogenetics studies, they pose particular complex issues to patients who must deal both with the risks and benefits related to the drugs they may be taking and the largely unspecified long-term research for which their donated sample will be used. In this situation Corrigan concludes that limits of consent have been exceeded and suggests that there is a real danger of individuals being exploited. The provision of greater levels of information, deemed by many as the answer to the failings of informed consent in practice is regarded as an unsatisfactory response. Corrigan calls for means of protecting research participants other than informed consent alone.

Klaus Hoeyer continues the critique of informed consent, developing in a different way Corrigan's discussion about the construction of certain kinds of personhood through the processes of informed consent. He presents evidence from empirical research he has undertaken on public participation in the Medical Biobank in Västerbotten. He compares the apparent lack of interest donors to this biobank have in the information provided to them when they agree to give a blood sample with the value that they place on being informed about the research during interviews he conducted with donors as part of his research. This paradox is addressed through a discussion of donors' perceptions of who should have responsibility for the conduct and consequences of genetic research. Hoeyer provides an analysis that embeds the practices of informed consent procedures in the specific social contexts of northern Sweden, and in the context of certain discourses of personhood that emerge through these procedures. He argues that the state in Sweden is posited as being uniquely able to exercise control over science through a number of measures, such as in the case of the biobank in Västerbotten a majority stake in UmanGenomics (a policy Hoeyer tells us was later rescinded). Interestingly, he finds that through their close identification with the state, individual donors conceive of themselves as sharing in the control supposedly exercised by the state. This conflation of state and individual is one that Hoeyer argues is particularly distinctive in northern Sweden. While the state is expected to take responsibility for science, Hoeyer explores how informed consent is an institutionalized practice by which individuals assume responsibility for themselves (rather than for the research and its implications as a whole) and so is performative of certain kinds of personhood. He discusses that sometimes donors attribute the blood they provide to the biobank as possessing qualities of their person, which is reinforced by the informed consent process, but at other times they depersonalize it, and see it as a resource that can be exploited for the benefit of the region. Hoeyer provides an engaging commentary of how blood moves across this terrain.

One particular aspect of genetic databases that has drawn comment is that they involve long-term, open-ended and multi-sited research to which individual participants are unable to give informed consent at the time of donating tissue samples and personal information (Lyttle 1997, Caulfield 2002). They also pose particular risks to participants, which comes not so much from the act of donation itself but from the future uses that could be made of genetic or personal information, which could give rise to invasion of privacy or discrimination both for the individual concerned and those to whom they are related. For these reasons Jane Kaye argues that the application of the principles of informed consent for medical research as established under international law cannot be so readily adopted in the context of genetic databases. Moreover, looking at the way the organizers of the Icelandic Health Sector Database claimed that under European law the project was exempt from the requirements of informed consent, because of the overwhelming public interest in the successful implementation and exploitation of this initiative, Kaye also denies exceptions to informed consent should apply. Given that private companies operate many genetic databases, Kaye questions whether as with epidemiological or public health research, these projects can be seen to be run in the public interest in quite the same way. Arguing for the abandonment of informed consent, she considers that a key question for policy is that of wider collective as well as individual interests of participants. Therefore, she proposes a number of measures that could be implemented such as community consultations involving patient groups or representatives, as well as measures to build public confidence such as independent ethical oversight and the establishment of trusts to hold and control information so as to ensure that public and commercial interests are balanced in the exploitation of genetic databases.

In chapter 8, Emma Williamson, Trudy Goodenough, Julie Kent and Richard Ashcroft address an issue current bioethics has tended to overlook: the perspectives of child participants in biomedical research. Their chapter focuses on proxy consent processes by which parents on behalf of their children agree to the long-term use of biological and genetic information for research. The context for this is the ALSPAC project in the southwest of Britain. As the authors remark, their research has been undertaken at a time when the status of children is changing as international agreements stress their rights and the importance of their voices in society. They examine the perspectives of children in the project in terms of their perceptions of the risks involved, and the influence they have over decision-making in relation to their parents. While recognizing that in practice decision-making is a shared process between parents and children, which the latter value and benefit from, the authors question the rights granted to parents within a proxy consent framework to take decisions about the long-term use of their children's data. This stems partly from the fact that childhood is by its nature a transitory period in life, but also perhaps more significantly from their findings that children and parents perceive what they consider to be sensitive information differently. This raises questions about whether current proxy consent frameworks best protect the interests of children. At the very least the authors argue that the views of children need to be integrated into the governance of these kinds of long-term projects that collect personal data to ensure their interests are indeed protected.

Notions of consent in relation to genetic databases have also been discussed more broadly than that of participants in existing research. Sue Weldon tackles the key question of wider public involvement in the actual setting-up of genetic databases and whether this should be conceptualized as a form of 'public consent' or more appropriately as a form of 'scientific citizenship'. Her chapter draws on various academic strands of social science research and is informed by current findings from an ongoing comparative study of the social, ethical and legal implications of population-based databases in the UK, Iceland, Estonia and Sweden. Weldon argues that while public participation in genetic databases is an issue requiring conventional ethical governance such as securing individuals' informed consent and ensuring that confidentiality and privacy are respected, these are highly individualistic concerns and that issues need to be framed in terms of a broader social terrain based on 'scientific citizenship'. Individuals encounter and participate in medical research within a social context and they engage at many levels implying a wider concept of engagement and another level of participation than that encompassed within the conventional mode of bioethics formulations. While the notion of the society or the social is part of a conventional bioethics frame insofar as individual rights are often weighed against duty to promote the 'common good', Weldon argues that what counts as the 'common good' is often assumed and she advocates instead that the public should be given an opportunity at the outset to negotiate what constitutes it.

The commercial context

In relation to many of the genetic databases we have mentioned in this introduction, such as the Icelandic Health Sector Database, UK Biobank or the Framingham Heart Study, the issue of commercial exploitation has been high on the agenda of many commentators (Barnett and Hinsliff 2001). This is part of a wider set of concerns articulated about the commodification of the human body, which has sparked a debate amongst legal scholars, ethicists, sociologists and others about the ownership of human tissue and genetic information (Dicks 1996, Witte and ten Have 1997, Nelkin and Andrews 1998, Knoppers 1999, Kennedy 2002, Laurie 2002, Parry 2003). Despite this focus the activities of the pharmaceutical, genomics or biotechnology industries to create genetic databases have tended to receive less attention (with the notable exception of Paul Martin (2001).

A notable contribution in this book to redress this situation is made by Graham Lewis, who examines the growing global commercial involvement of pharmaceutical and biotech industries in the collection and manipulation of human biological material. The activities of these industries are characterized by considerable secrecy presenting problems regarding claims about ethical standards and data security as commercial databases are not open to public scrutiny. Tissue collection and the construction of genetic databases is a rapidly changing field, both in terms of scale of activity and the type and sophistication of the information being extracted. Lewis identifies four sources of pharmaceutical industry collections: 'in-house' collections established by drug companies themselves; collections by intermediaries in the form of clinical genomics companies; existing public collections, such as hospital pathology collections, and other, research-based, tissue banks; and finally newly built public collections incorporating public health records and other personal information, such as the UK Biobank and the Icelandic Health Sector Database. The rapid expansion of tissue repositories and genetic databases of all types presents something of a policy dilemma for governments keen to encourage exploitation of new technologies whilst, at the same time, aware of the need to resolve public concerns surrounding genetic research and genetic databases. This chapter highlights some of the policy issues involved in the control and regulation of such databases. Lewis concludes that the challenge for governments is to encourage innovation in a manner that is ethically and socially acceptable. This requires, above all, public trust in the collection and operation of both tissue collections themselves and the genetic information derived from them.

In summary, the research presented in this book makes a much needed contribution that challenges existing frameworks and policies by highlighting the social and ethical contexts in which people participate in these new biomedical projects of the twenty-first century.

Notes

1. For some examples of policy-oriented discussions and guidelines adopted by national and international bodies in relation to the collection and storage of human tissue and genetic databases see Canadian Medical Research Council *et al.* (1998), Abbasi (2000), HGC (2000, 2002), Kaye and Martin (2000), WMA (2000), Berg (2001), Chadwick and Berg (2001), House of Lords (2001), Martin (2001), MRC (2001), Rumball and McCall-Smith (2001), Wilkinson and Coleman (2001), CIOMS (2002), Caulfield *et al.* (2003), Coriell Cell Repositories (2003).

2. As Ruth Chadwick and Kare Berg (2001) indicate, there are a number of antecedents to contemporary genetic databases in the form of disease or genetic registries, which were first created in the early twentieth century, and developed very much within the public health arena. These collections of medical and biological data tended to be small in scale. Advances in computing and bio-informatics associated with the Human Genome Project have been significant in allowing the emergence of large databases, holding and processing data on entire populations. For a historical account of clinical databases see Collen (1990), for discussions of sequencing databases and the impact of informatics see Doolittle (1997).

3. The literature indicates that there are numerous disease-specific databases in existence and there is a movement to harness the perceived power of databases of medical and genetic information to advance research on diseases such as cancer

(see for example Fenton and Sampson 1992, Chorru *et al.* 1994, MRC 2000, Teebi *et al.* 2002, Spinney 2003).

4. For accounts of developments associated with and issues raised by the Icelandic Health Sector Database see Enserink (1998), Andersen and Arnason (1999), Chadwick (1999), McInnis (1999), Kaye and Martin (2001), Rose (2001) and Meek (2002).

5. For discussions of the social, scientific and ethical issues by the UK Biobank see Coghlan (2000a, 2000b), Ho and Papadimitriou (2002), Wallace (2002), Stone and Vogel (2003) and Wilson (2003).

References

Abbasi, K. (2000). 'WMA to produce guidelines on health databases', *British Medical Journal* 320: 1295.

Abbott, A. (2001). 'Hopes of biotech interest spur Latvian population genetics', *Nature* 412: 468.

ALSPAC: Avon Longitudinal Study of Parents and Children (2003). Official website. Online. Available HTTP:
<http://www.alspac.bris.ac.uk/alspacext/index.shtm> (accessed 28 July 2003).

Andersen, B. and Arnason, E. (1999). 'Iceland's database is ethically questionable', *British Medical Journal* 318: 1565.

Annas, G.J. (2000). 'Rules for research on human genetic variation – lessons from Iceland', *New England Journal of Medicine* 342: 1830–1833.

Atkinson, W.I. (2000). 'The rush for the rock', *Globe and Mail*, Toronto, 5 January 2000. Online. Available HTTP:
<http://www.sfu.ca/-scoence/media/davidson.html> (accessed 7 October 2002).

Barbour, V. (2003). 'UK Biobank: a project in search of a protocol?', *The Lancet* 361: 1734–1738.

Barnett, A. and Hinsliff, G. (2001). 'Fury at plan to sell off DNA secrets', *Observer*, 23 September.

Berg, K. (2001). 'DNA sampling and banking in clinical genetics and genetic research', *New Genetics and Society* 20: 59–68.

Beskow, L., Burke, W., Merz, J., Barr, P., Terry, S., Penchaszadeh, V., Gostin, L., Gwinn, M. and Khoury, M. (2001). 'Informed consent for population-based research involving genetics', *Journal of the American Medical Association* 286 (18): 2315–2321.

Burton, B. (2002). 'Proposed genetic database on Tongans opposed', *British Medical Journal*, 324: 443.

Canadian Medical Research Council (MRC), the Natural Sciences and Engineering Research Council (NSERC), and the Social Sciences and Humanities Research Council (SSHRC) (1998). 'Ethical conduct for research involving humans'. Online. Available HTTP: <http://www.nserc.ca/programs/ethics/english/ethics-e.pdf> (accessed 1 May 2003).

Caulfield, T. (2002). 'Gene banks and blanket consent', *Nature Reviews: Genetics* 3 (8): 577.

Caulfield, T., Upshur, R.E. and Daar, A. (2003). 'DNA databanks and consent: a suggested policy option involving an authorization model', *BMC Medical Ethics* 4.

Chadwick, R. (1999). 'The Icelandic database – do modern times need modern sagas? *British Medical Journal* 319: 441–444.

Chadwick, R. and Berg, K. (2001). 'Solidarity and equity: new ethical frameworks for genetic databases', *Nature Reviews: Genetics* 2: 318–321.

Charru, A., Jeunemaitre, X., Soubrier, F., Corvol, P. and Chatellier, G. (1994). 'HYPERGENE: a clinical and genetic database for genetic analysis of human hypertension', *Journal of Hypertension* 12: S39–S46.

Chase, D. *et al.* (1997). 'North Cumbria Community Genetics Project', *Journal of Medical Genetics* 35: 413–416.

Coghlan, A. (2000a). 'A wild gene chase', *New Scientist* 2268: 16–17.

Coghlan, A. (2000b). 'Land of opportunity', *New Scientist* 2263: 31–33.

Collen, M.F. (1990). 'Clinical research databases – a historical review', *Journal of Medical Systems* 14: 323–344.

Connolly, A. (2000). 'Participants, experts discuss sale of Framingham data', *Boston Business Journal*, 18 August. Online. Available HTTP: <http://www.bozton.bizjournals.com> (accessed 7 May 2003).

Coriell Cell Repositories (2003). Policy for the Responsible Collection, Storage, and Research Use of Samples from Identified Populations for the NIGMS Human Genetic Cell Repository. Online. Available HTTP: <http://locus.umdnj.edu/> (accessed 28 July 2003).

Corrigan, O.P. (2003). 'Empty ethics: The problem with informed consent', *Sociology of Health and Illness* 25: 768–792.

Council for International Organizations of Medical Sciences (CIOMS) (2002). International Ethical Guidelines for Biomedical Research Involving Human Subjects. Geneva: CIOMS and WHO.

Cyranoski, D. (2000). 'Singapore to create nationwide disease database', *Nature* 407: 935.

deCODE Genetics (2003). Official website. Online. Available HTTP: <http://www.decode.com> (accessed 28 July 2003).

Dicks, D. (1996). 'Whose genes are they anyway?' *Nature* 381: 11–14.

Doolittle, R.F. (1997). 'Some reflections on the early days of sequence searching', *Journal of Molecular Medicine* 75: 238–241.

Enserink, M. (1998). 'Opponents criticize Iceland's database', *Science* 282: 859.

Estonian Genome Project (2003). Official website. Online. Available HTTP: <http://www.geenivaramu.ee/index.php?show=mainandlang=eng> (accessed 24 June 2003).

Fenton, I. and Sampson, J. (1992). 'A clinical and genetic database for management of familial adenomatous polyposis', *Journal of Medical Genetics* 29: 599.

Guillén, M., Lareu, M.V., Pestoni, C., Salas, A. and Carracedo, A. (2002). 'Ethical-legal problems of DNA databases in criminal investigation', *Journal of Medical Ethics* 26: 266–271.

Hagmann, M. (2000). 'UK plans major medical DNA database', *Science* 287: 1184.

Hansson, M. (2001). 'Introduction' to M. Hansson (ed.) *The Use of Human Biobanks: Ethical, Social, Economical and Legal Aspects*, Uppsala: Uppsala University.

Ho, Mae-Wan and Papadimitriou, N. (2002). 'Human DNA "biobank" worthless', *Institute of Science in Society*. Online. Available HTTP: <http://www.i-sis.org.uk> (accessed 28 July 2003).

House of Lords Select Committee on Science and Technology (2001). Human genetic databases: challenges and opportunities: with further evidence, House of Lords, Session 2000–01, 4th report, London: Stationery Office. 20-3-0001.

Human Genetics Commission (2000). 'Whose hands on your genes?' A discussion document on the storage, protection and use of personal genetic information. London: Human Genetics Commission.

Human Genetics Commission (2002). Inside information: balancing interests in the use of personal genetic data. London: Department of Health.

Husebekk, A., Iversen, O.-J., Langmark, F., Laerum, O., Ottersen, O. and Stoltenberg, C. (2003). 'Biobanks for health: optimising the use of European biobanks and health registries for research relevant to public health and combating disease', report and recommendations from an EU workshop held at Voksenåsen Hotel, Oslo 28–31 January 2003. Online. Available HTTP:<http://www.fhi.no> (accessed 26 January 2004).

Kaiser, J. (2002a). 'Population databases boom, from Iceland to the U.S', *Science* 298: 1158–1161.

Kaiser, J. (2002b). 'Private biobanks spark ethical concerns', *Science* 298: 1160.

Kaye, J. and Martin, P. (2000). 'Safeguards for research using large scale DNA collections', *British Medical Journal* 321: 1146–1149.

Kennedy, H. (2002). 'Bing's genes concern us all', *Guardian*, 22 May. Online. Available HTTP: <http://www.guardian.co.uk> (accessed 28 July 2003).

King, D. (2000). 'A democratic model for research using gene banks', written evidence submitted to House of Lords Science and Technology Committee, 29 September. Online. Available HTTP:
<http://www.parliament.the-stationery-office.co.uk/> (accessed 28 July 2003).

Knoppers, B.M. (1999). 'Status, sale and patenting of human genetic material: an international survey', *Nature Genetics* 22: 23–26.

Laage-Hellman, J. (2001). 'The industrial use of biobanks in Sweden: an overview', in M. Hansson (ed.) *The Use of Human Biobanks: Ethical, Social, Economical and Legal Aspects*, Report 1, Uppsala: Uppsala University.

Laurie, G. (2002). *Genetic Privacy, A Challenge to Medico-Legal Norms*, Cambridge: Cambridge University Press.

Lyttle, J. (1997). 'Is informed consent possible in the rapidly evolving world of DNA sampling?' *Canadian Medical Association Journal* 156: 257–258.

Marks, A. and Steinberg, K. (2002). 'The ethics of access to online genetic databases: private or public?' *American Journal of Pharmacogenomics* 2: 207–212.

Martin, P. (2000). 'The industrial development of human genetic databases', written evidence submitted to House of Lords Science and Technology Committee, October. Online. Available HTTP:
<http://www.parliament.the-stationery-office.co.uk/> (accessed 28 July 2003).

Martin, P. (2001). 'Genetic governance: the risks, oversight and regulation of genetic databases in the UK', *New Genetics and Society* 20: 157–184.

McInnis, M.G. (1999). 'The assent of a nation: genethics and Iceland', *Clinical Genetics* 55: 234–239.

McKie, R. (2000a). 'The gene map of Britain, and how it could save your life', *Observer*, 13 February: 16–17.

McKie, R. (2000b). 'The gene collector', *British Medical Journal* 321: 854.

Medical Research Council (MRC) (2000). 'The Medical Research Council announces funding for new genetic collections to study common diseases'. Online. Available HTTP: <http://www.mrc.ac.uk> (accessed 1 May 2003).

Medical Research Council (MRC) (2001). 'Human tissue and biological samples in research: operational and ethical guidelines', London: Medical Research Council (MRC).

Meek, J. (2000). 'Prospectors hunt human gene clues in New World', *Guardian*: London.

Meek, J. (2002). 'Decode was meant to save lives . . . now it's destroying them', *Guardian*, London.

Mieszkowski, K. (2003). 'Economic success is in the gene', *Guardian*, London.

Nature (1996). 'Editorial – gene donors' rights at risk', *Nature* 381: 1.

Nelkin, D. and Andrews, L. (1998). 'Homo economicus: commercialization of body tissue in the age of biotechnology', *Hastings Center Report*, September–October 1998: 30–39.

Nowak, R. (2000). 'Gene sale', *New Scientist*. Online. Available HTTP: <http://www.newscientist.com>.

Pálsson, G. (2002). 'The life of family trees and the book of Icelanders', *Medical Anthropology* 21: 337–367.

Parry, B.C. (2003). 'Bodily transactions: regulating a new space of flows in "bio-information"', in K. Verdery and C. Humphrey (eds) *Property in Question: Appropriation, Recognition and Value Transformation in the Global Economy*, Oxford: Berg Press, pp. 31–59.

Parry, B.C. (2004). *The Fate of the Collections: Exploring the Dynamics of Trade in Bio-Information*, New York: Columbia University Press.

POST: Parliamentary Office of Science and Technology (2002). 'The UK Biobank', Postnote 180, London: The Parliamentary Office of Science and Technology.

Rose, H. (2001). The Commodification of Bioinformation: The Icelandic Health Sector Database. Online. Available HTTP: <http://www.wellcome.ac.uk>, (accessed 26 January 2004).

Rumball, S. and McCall Smith, A. (2001). 'Draft Report on Collection, Treatment, Storage and Use of Genetic Data', SHS-503/01/CIB-8/3: UNESCO.

Sade, R.M. (2002). 'Research on stored biological samples is still research', *Archives of Internal Medicine* 162: 1439–1440.

Smaglik, P. (2000). 'Tissue donors use their influence in deal over gene patent terms', *Nature* 407: 821.

Spinney, L. (2003). 'UK launches tumor bank to match maligned Biobank', *Nature Medicine* 9 (5): 491.

Staples, S. (2000). 'Human resource: Newfoundland's 300-year-old genetic legacy has triggered a gold rush', *Business Magazine* 17 (3): 117–120.

Stone, R. and Vogel, G. (2003). 'UK biomedical agency gets a parliamentary tongue-lashing', *Science* 299: 1958–1959.

Teebi, A.S., Teebi, S.A., Porter, C. and Cuticchia, J. (2002). 'Arab Genetic Disease Database (AGDDB): a population-specific clinical and mutation database', *Human Mutation* 19: 615–621.

UK Biobank (2003). Online. Available HTTP: <http://www.ukbiobank.ac.uk> (accessed 28 July 2003).

UmanGenomics (2003). Official website. Online. Available HTTP: <http://www.umangenomics.com> (accessed 28 July 2003).

Unified Genome Database of Latvian Population (2003). Official website. Online. Available HTTP: <http://forum.europa.eu.int/irc/rtd/cogene/info/data/pub/Latvian%20Genome%20Project.htm> (accessed 28 July 2003).

Wallace, H. (2002). 'Biobank UK: is mental health a genetic problem?' Online. Available HTTP: <http://www.psychminded.co.uk/critical/biobank.htm>.

Wilkinson, J. and Coleman, R.A. (2001). 'The legal and ethical considerations relating to the supply and use of human tissue for biomedical research: a UK perspective', *Journal of Commercial Biotechnology* 8: 140–146.

Wilson, C. (2003). 'A healthy investment?' *New Scientist*, 10 May: 25.

Witte, J.I. and ten Have, H. (1997). 'Ownership of genetic material and information', *Social Science and Medicine* 45: 51–60.

WMA: World Medical Association (2000). 'The World Medical Association declaration on ethical considerations regarding health databases', October. Online. Available HTTP: <http://www.wma.net/e/policy/d1.htm>.

Chapter 2

Person, property and gift

Exploring languages of tissue donation to biomedical research

Richard Tutton

Introduction

Over the last decade the status and meaning of human tissue has become increasingly the focus of ethical, legal and sociological debates. This has happened at a time when its scientific and commercial value has grown with the emergence of population genetic databases, which are dependent on 'ordinary', 'healthy' people, with perhaps little direct interest in biomedical or genetic research, being willing to provide samples of their bodily tissue and personal information freely. To enrol these people into research projects of this nature, institutions have sought to bring participants into social relationships with researchers by emphasizing their common purpose in seeing improvements to human health. One way in which they have done this is to represent people's provision of tissue in terms of the ideals of social solidarity and personal altruism. In Britain this has been through powerful discourses of gift and 'gift-giving', and my purpose in this chapter is to explore the role that these discourses play in the way that human tissue is conceptualized and its use governed in the context of contemporary biomedical research.

A language of gift and 'gift-giving' has been used by those who resist what they see as the commodification of the human body to represent a non-exploitative relationship between the providers and users of tissue. The medical historian Susan Lawrence has argued for 'the firm denial of commodification [and to] seriously consider restricting research material to tissues and fluids that are the generous, unrestricted gifts of informed adults and their families' (Lawrence 1998: 133). Supporting the view that such material should be seen as altruistic gifts rather than commodities, the ethicist Suzanne Holland posits that 'our sense of dignity of humanity is fundamentally disturbed by the suggestion that which bears the marks of personhood can somehow be equated with property' (Holland 2001: 274). Those parts of the body that bear the 'marks of personhood' are those seen to be 'central to what characterizes living human persons, members of the human community' (Murray 1987: 37).[1] These include blood or organs that 'our social traditions suggest [. . .] may be given, but not sold' (Murray: 38). 'Gift-giving' is viewed as the only acceptable way for such parts of the body to be transferred because it accords respect for the dignity of the person involved (Canadian MRC *et al.* 1999). 'Gift-giving' is also conceived as altruistic in nature, as expressing a sense of community or solidarity, and performed to benefit the greater social good (Andrews and Nelkin 1998, Nelkin and Andrews 1998, Canadian MRC *et al.* 1999). An important contribution to this understanding of 'gift-giving' comes from the work of Richard Titmuss (1997) who examined the policies of blood donation over three decades ago. He saw the donation of blood as 'one of the most sensitive social indicators which, within limits is measurable, and one which tells us something about the quality of human relationships and of human values prevailing in society' (Titmuss 1997: 59). As this chapter shows, his account of voluntary blood donation as a 'gift relationship' remains a significant point of reference today in discussions about public participation, through the provision of tissue, in contemporary biomedical research.

I explore different languages of gift used in the British context to conceptualize the provision of tissue by individuals to biomedical researchers. My discussion will be based primarily on two examples of recent ethical guidelines on the use of human tissue. The first was produced by the Nuffield Council on Bioethics in 1995, as a direct response to the John Moore case; the other by the Medical Research Council (MRC) in 2001, developed during the period of the Alder Hey and Bristol Royal Infirmary incidents and the early proposals for UK Biobank. I should note how I intend to read these particular texts: Ulrich Beck (1997) has argued that 'questions of the political and economic "management" of risks actually or potentially utilized technologies' (Beck 1997: 19) have become increasingly significant in Western societies. Arguably, important tools in this 'management' are guidelines produced by scientific or ethical bodies that seek to regulate professionals' conduct and address perceived or communicated concerns of other groups such as government, commercial companies, special interests or the 'public-at-large'. Stephen Hilgartner (2000), for example, has explored the 'persuasive rhetoric' used by scientific advisory bodies in their guidelines to frame a particular problem and to define the boundary between science and politics. I read the MRC and Nuffield Council guidelines not only in the context of establishing a standard set of procedures for professionals, but also in terms of the substantial commercial interests in biomedical research and the perceived uncertainties amongst the 'public' about the governance of research.[2] Taken together, these guidelines are particular sites in which to explore the way that different languages of gift and 'gift relationships' are used in the production of 'boundary-work' (Gieryn 1983) around the commercialization of human tissue. I argue this has implications for who can and cannot financially benefit from and exercise control over its exploitation.[3]

Both sets of guidelines were produced by working groups of ethicists, legal scholars and medical professionals who considered many different types of human tissue provided and used for diverse purposes. However, in this chapter I am concerned only with biomedical research and the tissue most often provided and used for this purpose is blood, which of course is also given for transfusion purposes. To distinguish blood given for transfusion or other medical treatments and blood given for biomedical research I use the term tissue donation. The fact that the same substance is involved in both contexts is worth keeping in mind in the reading of this chapter (see Busby this volume). The different value blood has should also be appreciated: with regard to transfusion, blood is provided to someone else who may be experiencing a medical emergency, by contrast for biomedical researchers blood is only an efficacious way of extracting human DNA that subsequently becomes transformed in the processes of scientific knowledge production.

The chapter begins with a short account of Richard Titmuss' 'gift relationship' model, before turning to a discussion of the guidelines. I then discuss a critique of the continuing use of the language of gift with respect to tissue donation, which argues in favour of adopting a property paradigm to govern future relationships between users and providers. I also reflect a little on the interplay of the discourses of personhood and property, and of physical tissue, provided by individuals, and the genetic information derived from it.

Revisiting the 'gift relationship'

Titmuss' celebrated but also problematic concept of the 'gift relationship' emerged from his analysis of commercial and voluntary blood donor systems that operated in the 1960s (see Marshall 1973, Rose 1981, Oakley and Ashton 1997, Rapport and Maggs 2002). In essence he argued that the commercialization of blood donation led to the exploitation of poor and socially marginalized groups, the supply of high levels of contaminated blood, and diminished altruism and social solidarity. On the other hand, voluntary donor systems such as the one in Britain were much safer and fostered a sense of community because donors gave blood altruistically, knowing that 'their donations are for unnamed strangers without distinction of age, sex, medical condition, income, class, religion or ethnic group' (Titmuss 1997: 140). For Titmuss, one of the key human values that helped create the bonds of solidarity in modern industrial societies such as Britain was altruism (Rose 1981). It was a matter of public policy that institutions such as the National Health Service (NHS) should encourage altruistic behaviour.

Although Titmuss saw the 'gift relationship' as an exemplar of altruism he also saw that the viability of the donor system resided in the anonymity of that relationship because either donor or recipient could refuse to give or receive blood on 'religious, ethnic, political or other grounds' (Titmuss: 127). Therefore, it was imperative that donors relinquished control over the blood that they gave to the National Blood Transfusion Service, which had the responsibility of ensuring that the principles of social equality and equal access were maintained so as to keep the trust of donors and recipients. The state, therefore, played a central role in the 'gift relationship'.

As is well known, Titmuss drew on anthropological accounts of gift exchange to conceptualize voluntary blood donation. Marcel Mauss' (1997) argument that gift exchange was a key aspect of expressing and sustaining social solidarity provided an analogue for Titmuss' characterization of voluntary blood donation as constituting a set of social rather than economic relations outside of the market (Mauss 1997, see also Douglas 1997, Frow 1997).[4] Notably, Titmuss departed from Mauss' account by claiming that the British donor system was free of any obligations to give or reciprocate the 'blood gift'; people gave blood voluntarily from a sense of altruism without obligations, penalties or expectations of a return, and this was the closest in social reality to a 'free human gift'. Titmuss' denial of the obligation to reciprocate, at least in his characterization of the formal donor system, has led some critics to see his use of gift as tokenistic (Leach 1971, see also Douglas 1997, Frow 1997).[5] Others have pointed to how the welfare state cannot be considered a 'gift' domain because its forms of sociability do not involve the magical and dangerous ties of personal obligation, and that, 'in any strict sense the concept of the gift is irrelevant to the structural understanding of modern societies' (Frow 1996: 108).[6] Seeing the 'gift relationship' in terms of its representation of voluntary blood donation as an act of altruism that fosters greater social ties, it has achieved cultural, social, political and ethical resonance. It is a representation that still shapes the way that blood donation is viewed today, and commentators such as Susan Lawrence (1998), and Dorothy Nelkin and Lori Andrews (1998) have supported the idea of drawing on the conceptual and policy model of the 'gift relationship' for the governance of tissue donation to biomedical research.[7] It is how this model has been revisited in this latter context that I turn to now.

A new 'gift relationship' for a new genetics

Both the Nuffield Council and the MRC begin from a position that the commodification of the human body is undesirable, and draw support from international agreements such as the European Convention on Human Rights and Biomedicine that declares 'the human body and its parts shall not, as such, give rise to financial gain' (quoted in MRC 2001: 9). Specifically, they recommend that the provision of human tissue for research should not be regarded as a commercial transaction: 'research participants should never be offered any financial or material inducement to donate biological samples' (MRC 2001: 9). Instead, it is emphasized that the act of providing tissue is one of donation and that this 'clearly indicates what is involved is a gift' (Nuffield Council 1995: 68). As the MRC argues, this 'is preferable from a moral and ethical point of view, as it promotes the "gift relationship" between research participants and scientists, and underlines the altruistic motivation for participation in research' (MRC: 8).

The MRC guidelines use the language of 'gift relationship' to represent tissue donation as an altruistic enterprise that assists researchers to develop treatments and make scientific breakthroughs that will benefit human health. It is also implied that conceiving the relationship between 'research participants and scientists' – as recipients of the 'tissue gift' – in these terms will provide some kind of ethical and moral framework. However, this tissue 'gift relationship' is being proposed in a very different political, social and economic climate than at the time of Titmuss' evocation of the term. We are currently in a period of changing relationships between experts and lay people, public uncertainty about the outcomes of genetics research, and diminished confidence in medical institutions. Jane Kaye and Paul Martin (2000) note that, amongst other medically related incidents, the disclosures of tissue retention at various British hospitals has meant that 'public trust in the medical profession and the conduct of medical research has been seriously eroded' (Kaye and Martin 2000: 1146). Against this background, one can read the language of 'gift relationship' as recognizing the importance of establishing and maintaining public trust in medical professionals undertaking research.

Commercial involvement in research is another significant element to consider in this context. When the MRC and Wellcome Trust as funding partners behind UK Biobank commissioned market research into public attitudes on issues to do with this proposed project, it was reported that some respondents were ambivalent about the role of pharmaceutical companies. They perceived these companies as 'profit-driven', and voiced 'alarm' at commercial access to samples (Wellcome/MRC 2000: 6). Concern about public reaction to commercial involvement is expressed in the MRC guidelines:

> One of the major concerns in allowing commercial access to sample collections is the potential to damage the gift relationship between scientists and research participants. Research participants may be particularly sensitive to the idea of a company or an individual making a profit out of the tissue that they have freely donated.
>
> (MRC 2001: 12)

While both the MRC and Nuffield reject the commercialization of tissue provision, they state that diagnostics and therapies developed as a result of using such tissue in research is dependent on commercial involvement to ensure that they can be 'sufficiently available to benefit human health' (MRC 2001: 12). Such products require substantial long-term investment and 'will be best distributed through market structures' (Nuffield Council 1995: 52). Both sets of guidelines are based on a model of biomedical research that involves some kind of public–private partnership. Leading figures in the pharmaceutical industry have promoted the value of public–private collaborations. Robin Fears and George Poste (1999) at GlaxoSmithKline, for example, have suggested that private companies, universities, medical research charities and government should work together to establish a ' "third way" paradigm for clinical research' by creating 'pre-competitive public–private consortia' (Fears and Poste 1999: 268). Such a model permits what might be considered a politically acceptable way of utilizing the value of the UK NHS, a 'substantial but underused research resource [that] is probably the largest single source of medical information and well-characterized biological samples in Europe' (Fears and Poste 1999: 267), while avoiding public apprehension that commercial interests will dominate. UK Biobank is an example of a resource funded by and operated in the charitable and public sectors, but which will rely on in different respects commercial involvement and could have the potential to encourage future pre-competitive public–private collaborations.

To facilitate the commercial use of donated tissue, while addressing the kinds of concerns the public might have about this, it is proposed in the MRC guidelines that physical tissue samples will be stored by institutions designated as the formal recipients of these gifts: 'the MRC considers that it is more appropriate for formal responsibility for custodianship of sample collections to rest with institutions rather than with individual researchers' (MRC 2001: 12). This concurs with the conclusion of the Nuffield Council:

> If human tissue is procured by non-market procedures, while the products derived from human tissue may be manufactured and distributed by commercial organizations, there must be some intermediate institution, guided by professional codes and practices, which connects the market and the non-market structures.
>
> (Nuffield Council on Bioethics 1995: 53)

Such 'intermediate institutions' are named as universities and hospitals, which are charged with being the custodians of samples. It is anticipated that, along with ensuring research participants are told about commercial use as part of the informed consent procedure, such an arrangement will assuage potential public concerns over commercial exploitation by the private sector. Given their 'professional codes and practices', these institutions would therefore guarantee the ethical commercialization of genetic research; they would act in the public interest by allowing access by researchers on a non-exclusive basis so as to prevent the creation of effective monopolies over donated tissue.

This arrangement seems to be based on the premise that such institutions are indeed distinct from the commercial sector and do not themselves have commercial interests. Given the significant collaboration that now takes place across public and private sectors and the pressure on universities to develop the commercial applications of their research, this seems particularly problematic. This arrangement is also based on what both the Nuffield and the MRC note is a crucial difference between the physical tissue samples and the 'data or intellectual property derived from research using them' (MRC 2001:12). I go on to address this at length in the next section of this chapter, but in the interim it can be noted that this is key to understanding their position on the question of who can and cannot legitimately financially benefit from the exploitation of human tissue.

On this question both sets of guidelines have been influenced by the much-discussed judgement of the Supreme Court of California on the John Moore vs. Regents of the University of California case (1988–1990). These proceedings have been well-documented so I need not rehearse the background to them here (Boyle 1992, Frow 1997, Landecker 1999). After sections of his removed spleen were used to develop a cell line without his consent or knowledge, John Moore took legal action against the University of California at whose medical facilities he had been treated. One of his several causes of action involved a claim that he held a property right in the tissue used to grow the cell line, which entitled him to a share of any profits gained from its commercial exploitation. The Supreme Court denied this particular action. It reasoned that the tissue removed from Moore's body and the cell line were 'factually and legally distinct' (Boyle 1992: 1518), and that the tissue could not in itself be considered property, partly because it had not been invested with or altered by human labour. Instead it was a part of the 'commons' to which others may lay claim and transform into property through the process of human ingenuity and inventive effort (Frow 1997: 161).

In the cell line, the court did indeed see an example of human ingenuity and inventive effort and determined that, since Moore did not own the tissue removed from his body, he also had no claim over the cell line, thus no entitlement to a share of profits made from its commercial development. Moreover, the court concluded if the sources of tissue were to be granted property rights in human tissue, this would restrict the free exchange of biological materials and information amongst researchers and hinder future research. As James Boyle (1992) comments: 'to back up this argument the court painted a vivid picture of a vigorous, thriving public realm. Communally organized, altruistically motivated, and unhampered by nasty property claims, this world of research is moving dynamically towards new discoveries' (Boyle 1992:1432). Moore's property claim was 'a dangerous attempt to privatize th[is] public domain and to inhibit research' (Boyle 1992: 1519). While the court left open the question of whether the researchers could claim ownership of the tissue themselves, they had in any event already succeeded in patenting the cell line (Grubb 1998).

This case exemplifies the point made by the legal theorist Graeme Laurie (2002) that, 'while property rights are routinely granted in respect of human material, this is usually done to the exclusion of the one person who is central to the entire enterprise, namely, the individual from whom the material has been taken' (Laurie 2002: 304). Indeed, while the circumstances of the Moore case may have been exceptional, it has been a source of reference for regulatory, advisory and ethics bodies on the question of who can claim property rights in human tissue, including the Nuffield Council and MRC guidelines (see also Human Genetics Commission (HGC) 2000). I have noted that these guidelines reject the commercialization of tissue procurement and notions of ownership in relation to human tissue. The MRC, for example, prefers instead the term custodianship, which suggests possession rather than outright ownership. The UK House of Lords Science and Technology Committee's report on human genetic databases also concludes that: 'we do not regard ownership of biological samples as a particularly useful concept [. . .] we prefer the notion of partnership between participants and researchers for medical advance and the benefit of others' (House of Lords 2001).

From a legal perspective, Laurie argues that to conceive of donated tissue samples as gifts implies property and ownership rather than their absence, but also 'presumes the surrender of all residual interests in donated samples' (Laurie 2002: 317) by those who provide them. In claiming that donated tissue is a gift, the Nuffield Council conclude that it is 'free of all claims' (Nuffield Council 1995: 68) and that when a person voluntarily donates a sample they have 'not the slightest interest in making any claim to it once it is removed' (Nuffield Council 1995: 68). The MRC guidelines propose at the time of donation 'any property rights that the donor might have in their tissue would be transferred, together with the control over the use of the tissue, to the recipient of the gift' (MRC 2001: 8).

Given continuing legal ambiguity in Britain about whether there is property in human tissue, it is of note here that the MRC guidelines acknowledge donors may potentially have property rights, which they give up when they make their donation. The use of the term gift in this part of the guidelines could be read as having a specific legal meaning. In English Law gift is defined as

> The transfer of any property from one person to another gratuitously while the donor is alive and not in expectation of death. It is an act whereby something is voluntarily transferred from the true owner in possession to another person with the full intention that the thing shall not return to the donor.
>
> (Pettit 1993: 2)

Therefore, one may conclude that gift is used in this legal sense to describe the transfer of property, in other words the tissue sample from individual donors to the recipients. Its use delineates the boundary between who can and cannot make property claims and delimits the commercialization of human tissue in the context of biomedical research. The Nuffield guidelines note that donation does 'not ordinarily give rise to intellectual property rights' (Nuffield Council 1995: 74), and concludes that individuals who provide tissue samples are not in a position to claim an entitlement to any benefits arising from products developed using that tissue. The imperative that donors relinquish potential property rights in donated tissue permits commercial exploitation: the removal of one set of property claims from donors enables another set of claims by researchers over the various products created from the use of the samples involved.[8] This part of the guidelines reflects the legally binding provisions of the Convention on Biological Diversity (1992) and the GATT – TRIPs (General Agreement on Trade and Tariffs – Trade Related Intellectual Property Rights) Agreement (1994). As Margaret Lock (2002) relates, these agreements state that individuals surrender their property rights over tissue donated by them for research purposes unless special agreements have been signed to indicate otherwise. In this way, we have a sense in which guidelines made at a national level take into account the context of a global economy of biomedical research in which human tissue is increasingly valuable (see Lewis this volume).

But the issue is not only one of commercial exploitation it is also about control. To read this legalistic notion of gift as being a notable disjuncture from the language of the 'gift relationship' used earlier in the guidelines to emphasize altruism and solidarity is to overlook that Titmuss's model also entailed the surrendering of control over donated blood to the transfusion services. In effect, donors to research are being asked to do the same: to surrender control over their tissue samples to the institutions, the hospitals and universities, designated as the custodians of sample collections. For all intents and purposes, these kinds of institutions claim ownership over human tissue, even if the MRC prefers another term, which allows them to exercise that level of control over the use made of them.

In summary, the guidelines start from a position that disavows the commodification of the human body. Imbued with references to Titmuss' account of the 'gift relationship', there is a representation of tissue donation as a communal and altruistic realm in which researchers and research participants contribute to research that will benefit human health. The rhetoric of the 'gift relationship' and the organizational arrangements concerning the role of custodians creates both discursively and institutionally a boundary between the non-commercial domain of altruistic tissue donation and the commercial one of 'data or intellectual property'. It deflects attention away from the significant scientific and commercial interests that are at play and which both sets of guidelines are in fact concerned with facilitating in a way that excludes tissue providers and maximizes financial gain for tissue users. This is done through boundary-work that excludes physical tissue samples as property but allows the products derived from their use in research to be regarded as so. Moreover, by compelling donors to give up property rights in their bodily tissue, they are also unable to exercise any control over the research that is conducted or to stake a claim to any financial benefit accruing from the use of the tissue they provided.

This state of affairs has drawn the attention of legal theorists such as Graeme Laurie, to whose work I referred earlier, who argues for a rejection of the continued use of the language of gift and for the adoption of a new system of research governance based on property rights and increased participant control over their donated tissue. In the next part of this chapter I want to discuss this argument. In doing so I frame it in terms of the interplay of the discourses of personhood and property, and of human tissue and genetic information, which undergird the whole debate about tissue donation to research as discussed so far.

Between person and property: after the gift model?

I related at the start of the chapter that many academic commentators and ethical bodies have used the language of gift to frame their accounts of the use of human tissue in research to stress the values of dignity, altruism and solidarity, and to oppose the growing commodification of the human body and its parts. It is therefore allied with accounts of human tissue as being an inalienable part of human personhood rather than a commodity to be bought and sold. However, as I have shown in my reading of the guidelines, the language of gift in effect disrupts the boundary between person and property. Both the Nuffield Council and MRC texts conclude that the use of human tissue for research purposes should be governed according to a system of informed consent and the former is explicit in its rejection of a property model. However, the proposal that individuals may indeed have property rights in the samples they donate and that these rights are surrendered at the time of donation, seems to suppose that property could exist in personhood to the extent that these must be legislated for when drafting guidelines. In this way, these guidelines seem to operate with a degree of uncertainty about the status of human tissue, with the result of destabilizing that particular boundary between person and property that has been invested with such ethical significance.

The question of whether human tissue is person or property is one that has been addressed time and time again. Bartha Maria Knoppers (1995) suggests that genetic material should be considered *sui generis*, as neither person nor property, and to fashion rights and responsibilities of both tissue providers and users from this position. While Knoppers rejects the categories of person and property, Laurie seems to collapse them in his proposition that there is nothing in principle to prevent the recognition of property rights *in* aspects of human personhood (see also Grubb 1998).[9] He argues that the continuing use of the language of gift is an unsatisfactory response to the 'crisis of confidence' in medical research and posits that there is a public policy imperative for the implementation of a property model for the future governance of tissue donation to research. This would recognize what he calls the 'moral relationship' between 'individuality, personhood and body parts' (Laurie 2002: 318) that continues to exist after the moment when tissue is taken (see also HGC 2000). The premise of Laurie's argument is that the people who provide samples feel alienated from the way that research is conducted, and are distrustful of greater commercial involvement. They are 'undervalued, under-respected and undermined' (Laurie 2002: 309) by the current system of research governance. Continued public willingness to participate in research can only be ensured by giving them greater control over the uses made of the tissue they provide. Laurie proposes that only a system based on property rights, combined with established measures such as informed consent that protect autonomy, confidentiality and privacy, can achieve that goal.[10]

Laurie's argument is based on the distinction between small tissue samples given for research purposes and whole organs provided for transplantation. By restricting property rights to only the first category, the kinds of personal harm arising from a free market in organs could be avoided. Some support for this distinction can be taken from the Human Genetics Commission (HGC) who have asked whether a distinction can be drawn in principle between whole organs and small tissue samples that would 'justify allowing people to make profit from their tissues but not their organs?' (HGC 2000: 30). Even if we accepted this distinction, Titmuss' arguments against a commercial market in blood could still be rehearsed in relation to tissue samples: individuals who are poor or socially excluded may be driven by financial reward no matter how small to provide samples. This might not necessarily threaten their own lives nor those of others in terms of the transmission of disease as concerned Titmuss, but it could arguably produce social harm in the form of undermining altruism or what the HGC has called 'genetic solidarity' (HGC 2002).

While Laurie's argument collapses the distinction between personhood and property, the distinction between physical tissue samples and the information derived from them, also made in the MRC and Nuffield guidelines, remains problematic. He documents that under English Law there are no proprietary rights in abstract information not even when the individual is the source of that information. People may have a right to access information held about themselves, such as medical records, but this does not grant property rights in that information. Information can only be regarded as property when it has been involved in the process of inventive work, in which case it can be protected by intellectual property mechanisms such as patents. This situation is analogous to the relationship between excised bodily tissue that is not classed as property and the kinds of products created from that tissue such as cell lines that are protected as intellectual property. In expounding the argument for the recognition of property rights in tissue, Laurie finds the issue of whether those rights extend to cover the genetic information derived from them more problematic because by its very nature this is shared amongst people related to each other. Therefore, while in principle individuals could make a property claim in tissue removed from their bodies, including genetic information in that claim could be easily challenged by people to whom they are genetically related. At best, Laurie supposes that this could give rise to collective property claims.

It is of note that the focus of ethical concern in the guidelines is on the tissue itself, which is a finite resource that can diminish over time unless 'immortalized' in cell lines, rather than on the genetic information extracted from it, which becomes an infinite resource in its electronic form. This is partly a function of the fact that the authors of these sets of guidelines had to consider a number of different human tissues provided and used for varying therapeutic and research purposes. However, it is notable that neither set of guidelines addresses DNA or genetic information in terms of its ethical or scientific significance to participants or researchers. In terms of biomedical research, even for that which is not concerned exclusively with genetics, the value of human tissue lies not in the tissue itself but in the DNA or other molecules that can be extracted from it. This is recognized in terms of the intellectual property that might emerge from research using tissue, but it is not a part of the framework in which the discussion about the provision of human tissue for research is addressed. While the MRC and Nuffield Council concern themselves with the commodification of the human body, an editorial in *Nature* has suggested that the commodification of the genetic information it contains should also be of concern. It remarked that 'the implications of part of an individual's genetic identity being sold – that is, reduced to a commodity – flies in the face of many deeply held cultural beliefs of human value' (Nature 1996: 1).

In the United States, the activities of PXE International, a patient group formed for people with pseudoxanthoma elasticum (PXE) and their relatives, can be seen as an example of how a group of people with a genetic disorder have begun to exercise what could be argued to be in effect property rights over both physical tissue samples and forms of genetic information derived from both tissue and other sources (Smaglik 2000, Coghlan 2001, Fleischer 2001, Terry *et al.* 2001). PXE International negotiates and controls access by researchers to samples, family histories and other valuable data for research, as well as being named as co-author on scientific papers and patent applications. As such, the anthropologist Karen-Sue Taussig (in press) observes that PXE International is creating a new set of social relations in which 'ordinary people' are not just the 'containers of DNA' but are also co-producers of scientific knowledge. Although Taussig calls these people 'ordinary', the value of their DNA, and hence the basis on which PXE International exercises its control, resides precisely in the rarity of the condition. A different situation prevails when researchers investigate multifactorial diseases, because in a project such as UK Biobank they would be collecting tissue and other data from a more disparate general population, many of whom may be as yet unaffected by disease. Therefore, it is uncertain to what extent the 'PXE model' could be translated across different domains of public participation in biomedical research.

While other arguments could be considered against the adoption of a property model, one might ask whether the granting of property rights really would address what Laurie calls the 'crisis of confidence' in medical research?[11] To begin with, the depth and specificity of this 'crisis of confidence' in the governance of biomedical research could be questioned. A pubic consultation that was published by the Wellcome Trust and the MRC after publication of their proposals for UK Biobank in 2000 presents a complex picture with regard to this issue. It found that respondents considered the well-publicized incidents of organ and tissue retention at Alder Hey Hospital and Bristol Royal Infirmary and the case of Harold Shipman in the UK as exceptional events. There still seemed to be a great deal of trust in medical professionals and a belief in the positive benefits of medical research, although this varied amongst people of different age groups and experiences of disease. In terms of different groups or organizations trusted to use genetic information responsibly, a quantitative study commissioned by the UK HGC reported that general practitioners and the NHS scored very highly, while academic scientists scored 38 per cent and industrial scientists much less at 8 per cent (HGC 2000: 41). This could be taken to suggest that there is some ambivalence amongst respondents about individuals who are not directly involved in the therapeutic treatment or medical care of patients accessing genetic information.

The Wellcome/MRC consultation also revealed that most respondents imagined that people would donate samples out of a desire to help further research or to save other people's lives in the future. This is supported by a later consultation that discusses how respondents talked about participation in Biobank as a way of doing some 'good' (People Science and Policy 2002).[12] However, amongst some younger respondents, under the age of 30, there is some indication that the idea people should be paid for providing samples is acceptable and even desirable (Wellcome/MRC 2000). For the purposes of this current discussion, the problem is that little research has been done on public perceptions in terms of the debate about the ownership of human tissue. Therefore, there is little empirical evidence to illuminate Laurie's claim that a consent–property model would indeed secure greater public participation and confidence in research. Such research would usefully feed into the ethical and legal debates about the status and meaning of human tissue, and into the formation of policy guidelines by bodies such as the Nuffield Council or the MRC in the UK and their equivalents elsewhere in the world.

In the meantime, some developments associated with the UK Biobank are worth mentioning. While the language of gift is still part of the rhetoric used by the organizers of this project, the Interim Advisory Group, formed in February 2003 to develop ethical protocols for the handling of tissue and data, is considering measures that may provide a greater level of control for participants over their donated samples. First, participants will have the right to withdraw samples at any time without reason. Second, there are plans for the creation of an oversight body, the membership of which may very well include participants in UK Biobank. While there are practicalities relating to these arrangements to be considered, they could support the emergence of a different kind of relationship between researchers and participants by which it could become increasingly important to keep participants informed of, and their confidence in, the research process. The right to withdraw samples rather than to withdraw consent relating to them can be read as implying that participants have a de facto property relationship to both the samples and data they provide to this project.

Following this reading, participants, by retaining a right to withdraw at any time, will be in effect loaning rather than gifting their tissues samples to the project. The Biobank will be in possession of the samples and data to exploit them and control who has access to them according to the agreed terms of the informed consent procedure. However, participants can be seen to retain outright ownership by having the right to withdraw them at any time. In this way, the Biobank rather more than the intermediate institutions described in the MRC and Nuffield Council guidelines can be more accurately described as a 'custodian' of donated samples and data. At the time of writing I understand that the right of withdrawal would not extend to data that had been transformed into intellectual property as part of an inventive process, over which the researchers concerned would hold patents or other such protections. How the arrangements concerning the right to withdraw would be effected in practice remains to be seen. Notwithstanding these potential complications, together with the plans for an oversight body it is perhaps to be hoped that these arrangements will help create a different kind of relationship between researchers and participants in which participants have the potential to exercise greater control over the samples and data they provide. It will be a situation worth monitoring as ethical policies develop over the lifetime of UK Biobank.

Conclusion

The language of gift will no doubt continue to be a persuasive way in which institutions and researchers will speak about the donation of human tissue, precisely because of its connotations of altruism and the implication that individuals surrender control over it. As I suggested earlier in the chapter, the use of Titmuss' term 'gift relationship' should be seen as part of a move both by the MRC and more recently by the HGC to develop ways of representing the social contract between researchers and the public in the context of biomedical research. While the MRC has drawn rhetorically at least on the work of Titmuss, the HGC has developed the notions of 'genetic solidarity and altruism' (HGC 2002) that sees a shared human genome as meaning that people can help others by donating to research that will improve human health, and which either they or their descendants could benefit from in the future. Whether such attempts at representing a social contract between researchers and participants will resonate with participants and their own accounts of participation in biomedical research remains to be seen, and has been beyond the scope of this particular chapter to investigate (see Busby this volume, Hoeyer this volume, Hoeyer 2002, Tutton 2002). The development of UK Biobank is likely to be a significant site for academic inquiry into these questions over the next few years. As I suggested above, the gift model is perhaps already being challenged by the proposed arrangements relating to withdrawal of samples and data and participant oversight in UK Biobank.

On the question of the formation of ethical guidelines, there is a need to adopt a different approach to the question of how human tissue provided for research should be conceived and regulated. I have argued that the understanding in the MRC and Nuffield guidelines of what is gifted relates only to physical samples of human tissue provided by individuals and not the genetic information derived from that tissue, or any other kind of personal information that might be provided alongside the samples. This allows a boundary to be delineated between two economies, that of non-commercial tissue donation replete with a discourse of altruism, and the commercial domain of genetic information that can be transformed into intellectual property. This delimits the processes of commercialism in a way that insulates participants and their 'generous gifts' of samples from the activities of the commercial sector in biomedical research, with public bodies acting in a role of mediating those different domains. A more transparent approach to the development of guidelines is required, which would take into account both the specificities of the tissue and the fact that its scientific and commercial value lies in the genetic information derived from it. Such an approach would address the scientific and ethical meanings of human DNA or genetic information, which would undoubtedly impinge upon the discourses of personhood and property discussed in this chapter in novel ways, and work towards a new ethical practice.

Acknowledgements

Earlier drafts of this chapter were presented at the Centre for Family Research, University of Cambridge; Department of Social Studies of Medicine, McGill University; and Institute for the Study of Genetics and Biorisks in Society (IGBiS), University of Nottingham. I would like to thank everyone for their comments on those occasions, in particular Alberto Cambrosio, Janalyn Prest, Oonagh Corrigan, Bryn Williams-Jones, Martin Richards, Patrick Wallis and Paul Martin.

Notes

1. Other parts of the body, such as urine, fingernails or hair, are less central to the identification of the human person and so may more easily be sold for profit without a sense that personhood has been in any sense diminished (see also Nuffield Council 1995). The notion of dignity is an important aspect of the debate on the commodification of the human body. Rabinow (1999) notes that since the 'Preamble to the United Nations Charter declared its faith in the "dignity and value of the human person"' (Rabinow 1999: 103) in the aftermath of the Jewish Holocaust, 'dignity suddenly emerged as the a priori foundational principle of human existence' (Rabinow 1999: 103).

2. It is worth noting here that the MRC guidelines are applicable to all researchers who conduct or collaborate in research funded by the MRC. It is likely that both the MRC and Nuffield Council guidelines would be a source of reference in a court hearing on the legality of research practices (Kaye and Martin 2000).

3. Thomas Gieryn (1983) proposed the concept of boundary-work to describe the way that scientists attributed specific characteristics to science, its institutions and practitioners in order to construct a 'social boundary' between science and non-science. This boundary-work was analysed through particular rhetorical styles in which scientists 'describe science for the public and its political authorities . . . sometimes hoping to enlarge [their] material and symbolic resources . . . or to defend professional autonomy' (Gieryn 1983: 782).

4. Titmuss was not the first to see the potential relevance of gift exchange theory for the donation of human tissue – Renée Fox and Judith Swazey ([1967] 1978), noting the colloquial use of the term gift in medical, legal and popular discourses around organ donation, began to develop the term more systematically with reference to the anthropological literature.

5. A closer reading of Titmuss shows that he acknowledged the 'blood gift' cannot 'said to be characterized by complete, disinterested, spontaneous altruism. There must be some sense of obligation, approval and interest; some awareness of the need and of the purposes of the blood gift' (Titmuss 1997: 140). These are not effects of the formal organization of the donor system but originate informally in the wider social relationships in which donors lived.

6. Mauss also sought to argue that the reciprocity, co-operation and sociality between the state, employers and workers in the emerging welfare state of the twentieth century demonstrated that his theory of gift exchange was relevant to modern European societies (see Douglas 1997).

7. The conclusions of Titmuss' analysis of commercial and voluntary donor systems, especially in relation to safety issues, have informed governments' policies in the last quarter of the twentieth century. However, as Virginia Berridge (1997) points out, the appearance of HIV/AIDS in the 1980s revealed that the boundary between commercial and voluntary systems was highly misleading. 'Volunteer-fronted' systems in both Britain and France had 'become highly dependent on commercial sources' (Berridge 1997: 16) for the production of blood products (see Berridge 1997, Rabinow 1999).

8. It can also be noted that making the transfer of property rights an integral element of the donation of samples can be seen as an attempt to pre-empt a similar legal action to that of the John Moore case in Britain, especially since the

MRC guidelines would be a point of reference in any legal hearing. At the time of obtaining informed consent, the guidelines state that donors must be told who will be responsible for the custodianship of their sample and that 'their sample or products derived from it may be used by the commercial sector, and that they will not be entitled to a share of any profits that might ensue' (MRC 2001: 12).

9. Grubb (1998) argues that the existing informed consent regime, based on the maintenance of the integrity of the person, is inadequate because it relates only to the removal of tissue and not its subsequent use. Grubb proposes that individuals should be given certain – albeit limited – property rights to dispose of their tissue in the form of gift, sale or loan (see also Beyleveld and Brownsword 2000).

10. Laurie argues that the property model does not preclude the kind of altruistic-giving highlighted by the MRC guidelines and elsewhere and would not lead automatically to the practice of selling tissue samples (Laurie 2002: 309).

11. There are also arguments that property rights would hinder research, as the Supreme Court of California concluded in its judgement on the case of John Moore. For example, Warren Greenberg and Deborah Kamin (1993) say that human tissue is unlike other goods and services where economic efficiency is enhanced by their allocation to those who can afford to pay for them. The administrative costs that would arise from determining an appropriate value of a particular sample, especially when its commercial value downstream is uncertain, would outweigh that efficiency. When the commercial value of a sample could be judged prospectively, they do suggest a number of approaches for providing payment for (and in their view as a consequence grant a property right in) a sample, such as licensing agreements, tax credits or up-front one-off fees (Greenberg and Kamin 1993: 1075).

12. Although the main motivation for participation given by participants in this consultation was that of altruism, the authors of the report warn that this could be overemphasized in a group setting. Altruism is a socially powerful discourse with which people may identify in order to represent themselves to others as certain kinds of persons (see Busby this volume, Hoeyer 2002). As a concept altruism has been subject to philosophical scrutiny (see Rapport and Maggs 2002, Scott 2002), and research has indicated that lying behind people's accounts of their participation in various forms of tissue donation or research as 'altruistic' is a web of everyday social relationships, notions of obligations, reciprocity, community belonging and other personal life experiences (Fox and Swazey 1978, Titmuss 1997, Tutton 2002).

References

Andrews, L. and Nelkin, D. (1998). 'Whose body is it anyway? Disputes over body tissue in a biotechnology age', *The Lancet* 351: 53–57.

Beck, U. (1992). *The Risk Society: Towards a New Modernity*, Cambridge: Polity Press.

Berridge, V. (1997). 'AIDS and the gift relationship in the UK', in A. Oakley and J. Ashton (eds) *The Gift Relationship, From Human Blood to Social Policy*, London: London School of Economics and Political Science.

Beyleveld, D. and Brownsword, R. (2000). 'My body, my body parts, my property?' *Health Care Analysis* 8: 87–99.

Boyle, J. (1992). 'A theory of information, copyright, spleens. Blackmail and insider trading', *California Law Review* 80: 1415–1540.

Canadian Medical Research Council (MRC), the Natural Sciences and Engineering Research Council (NSERC), and the Social Sciences and Humanities Research Council (SSHRC) (1998). Ethical conduct for research involving humans'. Online. Available HTTP: <http://www.nserc.ca/programs/ethics/english/ethics-e.pdf> (accessed 1 May 2003).

Coghlan, A. (2001). 'Patient power', NewScientist.com. Online. Available HTTP: <http://www.newscientist.com/news/news.jsp?id=ns9999448> (accessed 1 May 2003).

Douglas, M. (1997). 'No free gifts', in M. Mauss (ed.) *The Gift, The Form and Reason for Exchange in Archaic Societies*, trans. W.D. Halls, London: Routledge.

Fears, R. and Poste, G. (1999). 'Building population genetics using the UK NHS', *Science* 284: 267–268.

Fleischer, M. (2001). 'Seeking rights to crucial gene: parents of children with PXE took steps to control samples used in research for a cure', *National Law Journal* 23 (44): C1.

Fox, R.C. and Swazey, J. (1978). *The Courage to Fail: A Social View of Organ Transplants and Dialysis*, London: University of Chicago Press.

Frow, J. (1996). 'Information as gift and commodity', *New Left Review* 219: 89–108.

Frow, J. (1997). *Time and Commodity Culture, Essays in Cultural Theory and Postmodernity*, Oxford: Clarendon Press.

Gieryn, T. (1983). 'Boundary-work and the demarcation of science from non-science: strains and interests in professional ideologies of scientists', *American Sociological Review* 48: 781–795.

Greenberg, W. and Kamin, D. (1993). 'Property rights and payment to patients for cell lines derived from human tissues: an economic analysis', *Social Science and Medicine* 36 (8): 1071–1076.

Grubb, A. (1998). '"I, me, mine": bodies, parts and property', *Medical Law International* 3: 299–317.

Hilgartner, S. (2000). *Science on Stage: Expert Advice as Public Drama*, Stanford: Stanford University Press.

Hoeyer, K. (2002). 'Conflicting notions of personhood in genetic research', *Anthropology Today* 18 (5): 9–13.

Holland, S. (2001). 'Contested commodities at both ends of life: buying and selling gametes, embryos, and body tissues', *Kennedy Institute of Ethics Journal* 11: 263–284.

House of Lords Select Committee on Science and Technology (2001). Human genetic databases: challenges and opportunities, House of Lords, Session 2000–01, 4th report, London: Stationery Office.

Human Genetics Commission (2000). 'Whose hands on your genes?' A discussion document on the storage, protection and use of personal genetic information, London: Department of Health.

Human Genetics Commission (2001). 'Public attitudes to human genetic information: People's panel quantitative study', London: Department of Health.

Human Genetics Commission (2002). 'Inside information: Balancing interests in the use of personal genetic data', London: Department of Health.

Kaye, J. and Martin, P. (2000). 'Safeguards for research using large scale DNA collections', *British Medical Journal* 321: 1146–1149.

Knoppers, B.M. (1995). 'Human genetic material: commodity or gift?' in R. Weir (ed.) *Stored Tissue Samples: Ethical, Legal and Public Policy Implications*, Iowa City: Iowa University Press.

Landecker, H. (1999). 'Between beneficence and chattel: the human biological in law and science', *Science in Context* 12: 203–225.

Laurie, G. (2002). *Genetic Privacy, A Challenge to Medico-Legal Norms*, Cambridge: Cambridge University Press.

Lawrence, S.C. (1998). 'Beyond the grave – the use and meaning of human body parts: a historical introduction', in R. Weir (ed.) *Stored Tissue Samples: Ethical, Legal and Public Policy Implications*, Iowa City: Iowa University Press.

Leach, E. (1971). 'The heart of the matter', *New Society* 17(434): 114–115.

Lock, M. (2002). 'The alienation of body tissue and the biopolitics of immortalized cell lines', in N. Scheper-Hughes and L. Wacquant (eds) *Commodifying Bodies*, London: Sage.

Marshall, R.M. (1973). 'An appreciation – Richard M Titmuss', *British Journal of Sociology* 24: 137–139.

Mauss, M. ([1925] 1997). *The Gift, The Form and Reason for Exchange in Archaic Societies*, trans. W.D. Halls, London: Routledge.

Medical Research Council (MRC) (2001). 'Human tissue and biological samples for use in research', April 2001, London: Medical Research Council.

Murray, T.H. (1987). 'Gifts of the body and the needs of strangers', *Hastings Law Center Report*, April 1987: 30–38.

Nature (1996). Editorial – 'Gene donors' rights at risk', *Nature* 381: 1.

Nelkin, D. and Andrews, L. (1998). 'Homo economicus: commercialisation of body tissue in the age of biotechnology', *Hastings Center Report*, September–October 1998: 30–39.

Nuffield Council on Bioethics (1995). 'Human tissue: ethical and legal issues'. Online. Available HTTP: <http://www.nuffieldfoundation.org/bioethics> (accessed 1 May 2003).

Oakley, A. and Ashton, J. (eds) (1997). 'Introduction to the new edition', in *The Gift Relationship, From Human Blood to Social Policy*, London: London School of Economics and Political Science.

People Science and Policy Ltd (2002). 'Biobank UK: a question of trust: A consultation exploring and addressing questions of public trust'. Online. Available HTTP: <http://www.ukbiobank.ac.uk/documents/consultation.pdf> (accessed 1 May 2003).

Pettit, P.H. (1993). 'Gifts inter vivos', in Lord Hailsham (ed.) *Halsbury's Laws of England*, 20, London: Butterworths.

Rabinow, P. (1999). *French DNA: Trouble in Purgatory*, London: University of Chicago Press.

Rapport, F.L. and Maggs, C.J. (2002). 'Titmuss and the gift relationship: altruism revisited', *Journal of Advanced Nursing* 40 (5): 495–503.

Rose, H. (1981). 'Re-reading Titmuss: the sexual division of welfare', *Journal of Social Policy* 10(4): 477–502.

Scott, N. (2002). 'Eugenics perpetrated through altruism', *Science as Culture* 11 (4): 505–522.

Smaglik, P. (2000). 'Tissue donors use their influence in deal over gene patent terms', *Nature* 407: 821.

Taussig, K.S. (in press). 'Molecules, medicine and bodies: building social relations for a molecular revolution in medicine', in S. McKinnon and S. Silverman (eds) *Complexities: Anthropological Challenges to Reductive Accounts of Biology*, Chicago: University of Chicago Press.

Terry, P.F., Terry, S.F., Marais, A.S., Pasquali-Roncheti, I., Boyd, C., Johnson, E., Le Roux, T. and Bercovitch, L. (2001). 'Effective international collaboration in rare disease research', *American Journal of Human Genetics* 69 (4): 382.

Titmuss, R. ([1970] 1997). *The Gift Relationship, From Human Blood to Social Policy*, A. Oakley and J. Ashton (eds) London: London School of Economics and Political Science.

Tutton, R. (2002). 'Gift relationships in genetic research', *Science as Culture* 11 (4): 523–542.

Wellcome Trust/MRC (2000). 'Public perceptions of the collection of human biological samples'. Online. Available HTTP: <http://www.ukbiobank.ac.uk/documents/perceptions.pdf> (accessed 1 May 2003).

Chapter 3

Blood donation for genetic research

What can we learn from donors' narratives?

Helen Busby

Introduction

Regulation of the donation of body tissue for research has recently become the subject of intense scrutiny in the UK. Concern has been expressed about the impact of a number of controversial developments in medicine and in biotechnologies generally on the willingness of people to participate in ongoing research. If the practitioners and institutions of science are being pushed to confront their dependence on the support of the communities which fund them, the situation faced by genetic research is particularly striking. To date, much of the genetic research directly involving human subjects has been concerned with particular, often rare, genetic diseases and has sought the participation of affected patients and their relatives. The current agenda envisages a phase of larger population-based studies to explore the genetic contribution to common diseases and to adverse drug reactions.[1] Thus a wave of larger studies is anticipated, seeking the involvement of many thousands of people who have no prior experience of or interest in a particular disease.

In Britain, in particular, cohort studies are planned to explore the role of genetic factors in the development of common diseases (Berger, 2001). The proposed UK Biobank, a large-scale collection and database of genetic, environmental and lifestyle information, is perhaps the most dramatic and well-reported development. Funded by the UK's Medical Research Council (MRC) and Department of Health together with the Wellcome Trust, a medical research charity, this project seeks to be the largest databank of its kind in the world. As highlighted in the previous chapter, such new initiatives have been greeted by a wave of consultations with the public and professionals, policy discussions and inquiries, in which the ethical issues involved and the regulatory frameworks which might be applied to these new developments are explored and elaborated.[2] The importance of public trust features centrally in the discussions about these shifts in the way that research is organized. Indeed these developments have highlighted the way in which the trust generally associated with the NHS can be an important resource for research. Other recurring themes in the discussions include the reliance on informed consent as a linchpin of protection for research subjects, and the emphasis on privacy as a central concern, both of these occurring in a wide range of contexts and disciplines.

Following Raymond Apthorpe, a starting point for this chapter is the importance of 'the language and writing of policy and research [in functioning as] a type of power' (Apthorpe 1997: 43). Keywords and concepts are seen as having accumulated meanings historically, some of these becoming metaphors which underpin policy. Each organizing concept will shape the discussion in one way, inevitably shifting attention from other aspects of the phenomenon. As discussed by Richard Tutton (this volume), the conceptualization of tissue donation in this context as a 'gift' is one such prominent organizing concept. A number of powerful and sometimes contradictory concepts co-exist under this heading. In more general clinical parlance, organ and tissue donations are often referred to as a 'gift of life' by some of those involved in organ trans-plants (Simmons *et al.* 1987). The way in which such rhetoric may obscure the realities of living and of dying for both the donor and the recipient has been criticized by a number of sociologists (Fox and Swazey 1992). In relation to blood donation, the donation of blood as a 'gift to strangers' with important moral and social dimensions is a powerful image, pioneered by Richard Titmuss' ([1970] 1997) classic study, and continues to be highly influential in both policy and clinical discourses. More particularly, in recent policy and clinical discussions about genetic research, the notion of tissue donation as a gift seems tied to questions of ownership of tissue: if tissue is 'gifted', it becomes the property of the recipient for legal purposes, thus resolving a number of tricky legal questions about ownership of such tissue (see Tutton this volume). Despite the slipperiness of the idea of 'the gift' in this context, and the diverging ways in which such a concept is used, it is used so frequently and tenaciously that we may point to it as a key mobilizing metaphor.

A feature of much of the discussion about people's involvement as volunteers in genetic research is that it has been dominated by abstract theories, whether derived from law, bioethics or (indirectly) from anthropology.[3] Until recently, there has been relatively little empirical work in this context (see Haimes and Whong-Barr this volume, Williamson *et al.* this volume). The study of local sites of participation in research may contribute to an unsettling of these theories and begin to delineate more specific problems to be addressed at these sites. This chapter begins with a review of some of these analytical concepts, which are of course more textured than the broad brush strokes above suggest. I then move on to outline and refer to two 'case studies' of different kinds of blood donation. The first of these is the case of 'ordinary' blood donors at one site in the UK, the second is with donors of blood for a particular genetic research project, who did not have a prior concern with a disease designated as having a genetic cause. Some of the issues emerging from the case of 'ordinary' blood donors are outlined, and these foreshadow a more detailed discussion of donation for the genetic research project. A discussion of the dynamics of knowledge and trust in these particular contexts is used to interrogate some of the prevailing assumptions.

Interrogating analytical frameworks

Non-maleficence, beneficence, autonomy and justice: these principles have become guiding principles in contemporary bioethics. However, one of these – 'autonomy' – has become singularly prominent in the practice of bioethics (Dingwall 2002). Within applied ethics the obtaining of individual informed consent has by and large been seen as the way to operationalize that principle. Partly as a consequence of the emphasis on autonomy, questions about the distribution of healthcare, and about public health have been 'pushed to the margin in much of bioethics' (O'Neill 2002: 4). The emphasis on autonomy, its social and political underpinnings and cultural resonances, has not gone unquestioned in recent years; there are articulate critiques both within and beyond bioethics (Frank 2000). Amongst these, Ruth Chadwick and Kare Berg (2001) call for a shift towards solidarity and equity as a framework for considering larger scale genetic research (Chadwick and Berg 2001: 320). The argument here is based on the potential for research to benefit the whole community – as opposed to only those affected by a particular disease, as is often the case with particular drug trials for instance – combined with the necessity for valid epidemiological research to include representatives from a wider population. Despite the recent discursive turn in bioethics, however, the institutions which are mandated to undertake the quasi-regulatory role of ethics – such as medical research ethics committees – are constituted with reference to the more established principles mentioned above.

Within sociology, the social issues relating to the development of new medical technologies have been explored mainly through two strands of work: the field of Science and Technology Studies (STS) and the Sociology of Health and Illness. Both have been deeply concerned with the problems of differential expertise in relation to technologies.[4] A significant development within both traditions is the elaboration of concepts of lay 'epidemiology', 'knowledge' or 'expertise' to interpret the ways in which lay people mobilize resources, and to challenge fixed ideas about lay people's lack of power in relation to medicalization (Davison *et al.* 1991, Wynne 1991, Williams and Popay 1994). In the course of the development of both traditions of work, the dichotomy between lay and expert knowledge has been challenged. For example, Jeanette Edwards does this by underlining the extent to which scientists use lay knowledge in contexts outside their own expertise (Edwards 1999). Some have gone as far as to call the concept of lay expertise an oxymoron, and argue instead for the use of the term 'experience-based experts':

> We say that those referred to by some other analysts as 'lay experts' are just plain experts – albeit that their expertise has not been recognized

by certification; crucially, they are not spread throughout the population, but are found in small specialist groups.

(Collins and Evans 2002: 238)

Notwithstanding the subtleties of these debates, the concept of lay knowledge or expertise remains prominent in the literature about those facing environmental or medical controversies. This is in part because of the alliance of the concept (of lay knowledge) with a political drive to recognize the agency of those who were formerly seen as passive in the face of technical experts.

Much of the work on the social context of developments in genetics echoes wider theoretical discussions about a 'risk society' (Beck 1992). The theorizing of trust holds a pivotal place in these discussions, with the erosion of trust in expert authorities or systems often being postulated (Giddens 1990). Such theories have become highly influential both in academic debates and in UK government science policies. However, the proponents of such overarching theories about trust have been criticized for a lack of empirical grounding or testing. More recent work tends to question these overarching theories and to point to a greater diversity of relationships with 'risk' (Elliott 2002, Lupton and Tulloch 2002). In seeking to analyse specific local contexts for the dynamics of some such relationships, the work described below builds on these critiques.

Donating blood for transfusion and other medical treatment

In contrast to genetic techniques and research, blood donation and transfusion are widely accepted health technologies. As blood is the most commonly requested tissue for (epidemiological) genetic research, the perspectives of blood donors can provide a reference point for thinking about genetic donors. Widely lauded as 'altruistic', their individual characteristics, motives, personalities and behaviours have long been of interest to psychologists (see for example Piliavin 1990). But there is a sense in which social arrangements construct donors, and it is these that are my primary concern.

There is another important sense in which blood donation is a point of reference for the debate on genetic donation: Richard Titmuss' work on 'gift relationships' in which he proposed a concept of blood donation as a 'gift to strangers' with a moral dimension has been hugely influential in both academic work and more recently in policy discussions about tissue donation for genetic research (Titmuss [1970] 1997, Robinson and Murray 1999, MRC 2001, People, Science and Policy Ltd 2002, Tutton 2002). Titmuss' concept of blood donation as a 'gift to strangers' has been invoked in the context of the UK Biobank, in which samples will be sought from the general population.

The host of the first case study, the UK's National Blood Service (NBS), was set up in 1993 to take over from the services previously run by regional health authorities. The NBS is now a special health authority charged with the collection, screening and supplying of blood and blood products to the NHS, and with research and development in this field. The NBS employs thousands of donor carers to carry out the day-to-day work of caring for donors and taking blood, mostly at community centres and churches throughout the country. Each region also has one or more permanent sites, where donors can drop in on any weekday and give blood without an appointment. With a few exceptions, interviews with blood donors took place at one such site in a metropolitan area of the north of England. Interviews were undertaken by the author after donors had given blood, alongside the rest area where hot drinks and biscuits are provided.

One hundred short interviews were conducted for this research, of approximately equal numbers of men and women, ranging in age from 18 to late 60s, but with most being in their 30s, 40s and 50s. These interviews sought to explore the dynamics of decision-making for NBS donors, any concerns they might have about the procedures involved and their views about the uses to which blood may be put. In addition they aimed to explore how these NBS donors might view the possibility of donated blood being used for research, and in particular for genetic research. To this interview data was added fieldnotes from observation of the donor sessions: these observations counter the emphasis on verbal accounts to some extent, reminding us that giving blood is a physical process in which donors are cared for in a variety of tacit and explicit ways.

The place of work and family were prominent in the reasons or triggers for beginning to give blood, and indeed in people's narratives more generally. When talking about the rationale or motivation for donating blood, many talked in fairly general terms about blood donation being worthwhile or a good thing to do for others. Some referred to a general perception of blood being needed, some to awareness of need in the present or past by a family member, and a smaller number to a response to an NBS appeal for donors in this context. There is some consistency in these interviews about the views of donors on blood donation as a social arrangement. Essentially, most donors express the view that donating blood is a donation to a 'bank' which they themselves, their relatives or strangers can draw on. Whilst this may at first appear a self-evident statement, it contrasts with some common notions about blood donation as being motivated by 'pure altruism'. For these blood donors, donation is seen in quite a practical light. As people get older they are more likely to know someone who has needed blood in difficult circumstances, and if they have not, the NBS promotional campaigns are likely to draw to their attention the need for blood in the lives of those whom they know. Recipients of blood donation can still give blood in many circumstances, and often do. Donors perceive themselves and their families as potential recipients in a direct sense. Some donors view the blood screening and care given at the centre as a health check in itself. Thus for many donors their view of the act of blood donation contains a recognition of reciprocity both in terms of possible drawings out in the future from the blood 'bank', and in terms of a moral economy where a feeling of doing good is of value in itself.

Dynamics of knowledge and trust

Blood donors' accounts often seemed on the face of it very straightforward, indicating a kind of catch-all trust or even lack of interest with what would be done with the blood. For example, one donor said: 'As I see it once it comes out of here and into their hands they can do with it what the hell they want, I've done my bit.' My questions about any concerns or worries about giving blood were often met with a blank dismissal. When asked about the uses to which the blood is put, donors were sometimes puzzled or alternatively embarrassed at their lack of detailed knowledge. NBS policies allow for the possibility that donated blood may be used for research purposes. More recently this has been indicated on the donor consent/declaration form. However only a handful of donors mentioned research when asked about the uses to which the blood was put: there seemed to be a disjuncture between donors' formal consent, as indicated on the signed declaration, and the uses for the blood which were prominent in their explanations to me, such as use in operations and other such emergencies.

There are a number of ways of looking at these dynamics of knowledge. It is important to consider these in the context of the self-evident but over-looked one of blood donation: in this process, donors are cared for in many tacit ways, whilst they hand over blood and indeed the responsibility for its use. The trust here is not built on detailed knowledge or on verbal interaction, but rather on a physical and practical relationship with the donor carers and the donor centre itself. Because few donors expressed dissatisfaction with the level of information, indeed rather the opposite, we might see the arrangement as fit for purpose in this particular case. We might see this as a part of a wider phenomenon of 'informed compliance' (Stapleton *et al.* 2002), where patients or donors have sufficient information to enable them to comply with the essential tasks which they undertake, in this case primarily detailed informa-tion on 'do's' and 'don'ts' before and after giving blood. There are a number of ways of thinking about these accounts and what these perspectives bring to bear on the nature of consent in this context. These are discussed further below.

When asked about their views on the use of blood for research in principle, an overarching theme from the interviewees as a group was a statement of confidence in the importance and necessity of research with reference usually being made explicitly to its part in progressing medical knowledge. Trust was significant, even palpable in this context. There was a sense in which donors, working at the limits of their expertise, chose to hand over trust, a choice with physical and emotional dimensions as well as the more evident cognitive element. The paradox is that whilst we appear to have an only partially informed consent for the uses which are made of the blood donation, the contract between organization and donor is seen by most as having a sustainable moral basis. In the case of the NBS, the practical reciprocity of a donation which is seen to have potential and tangible benefits to oneself, one's family and friends and other 'strangers' is widely seen as the underlying basis of the arrangement.

Practical reciprocity, the dynamics of knowledge and trust, and the embeddedness of these issues within the contexts of work and family thus emerged as sensitizing themes for the undertaking of interviews with genetic donors.

Donating blood for a genetic research project

For the second case study, donors were selected from a genetic research project based in a research unit at a university hospital in a large city, likewise in the North of England. An important criterion for the selection of this research site was that it enabled access to people being asked to participate in genetic research who did not have a prior interest or involvement in a 'genetic' disease.[5] The university and NHS bodies have well-established regional services in clinical genetics and allied research activity. Nevertheless, the predominant research activities in the area remain the study of rarer diseases, in which there is often a substantial overlap of clinician/researcher roles. The unit undertook this kind of research, but is also a leading site for the development of epidemiological genetic research in its field. The unit and its donors are not necessarily 'representative' of genetic research activity and donation; indeed in the absence of a national register for such activity it would be difficult to know how representativeness could be ascertained. The project selected was a study of psoriatic arthritis, a disease affecting both skin and joints, for which the aetiology is uncertain: the unit's research was concerned with identifying the extent to which there *may* be a genetic component.

The unit recruits volunteers for this project nationally by several means, including advertisement in local newspapers and referral by hospital consultants. Inclusion criteria for this particular study were a diagnosis of arthritis and of psoriasis, or of psoriatic arthritis. Following confirmation of this diagnosis, volunteers are visited by a research nurse from the unit, who undertakes a clinical examination, may take a photograph of the psoriasis, and administers questionnaires on health status, pain and disability. Data on family history of both skin and joint problems are taken, and agreement is sought for access to NHS records for this study if required. Finally a blood sample is taken: the consent form states that the blood is 'gifted to the unit' for research purposes, also that it may be used by other research laboratories working (only) on arthritis/psoriasis. The form states that no genetic data will be fed back to participants.

Twenty-seven interviews were undertaken with donors recruited by these means, 14 of these being women and 13 men, ranging in age from their 20s to their 60s. In interviews with these donors, the aim was to explore the ways in which people had become involved in the genetic research project. When asking them why they had agreed to participate, I wanted to learn more about how they think about their interest in the blood which is donated, and I was interested in what (if anything) was special about giving blood for genetic research. I was generally interested in how people talked about this blood donation for genetic research. I asked them too about the condition itself and the ways in which it affected their lives. In relation to the genetic study itself, I asked people to tell me about the information they received and whether they had any worries or concerns about the study; I wanted to elicit whether the genetic element of the study featured here.

Most of the interviewees indicated that they were happy to help contribute to research for a condition which had caused them some degree of suffering or inconvenience, and that by doing so they hoped to contribute to knowledge about and treatment for the condition. For some the initial comment about participation in the study was framed more in terms of having been asked and 'not minding'. A few indicated that sympathy or liking for the researcher or for a particular consultant was a factor. Two study participants were evidently looking for and expecting specific feedback on genetic tests (which would not be available to them under the terms of this study) and were disappointed to find that this was not to be forthcoming.

Informed consent and the dynamics of knowledge

The obtaining of informed consent has conventionally been considered a linchpin of research ethics (see Corrigan this volume). In this case study I found that initial consideration of whether or not participants could be considered to have given informed consent specifically to the analysis of their DNA disclosed some ambiguity. I shall take three examples from interviews to illustrate this unfolding ambiguity. Mrs Burnett works as a nurse in the NHS and it was clear that her knowledge of the health system, including previous exposure to research projects through her work, was brought to bear on this study: 'I've got enough knowledge not to be scared of anything'. There was a clear sense that she had understood the nature of the study at the outset, in particular that she did not expect any benefit from the research, that she understood there would be no feedback of the results of DNA analysis to herself, and the nature of research as a long-term process. When probed about the use of DNA in the study she initially responded that 'to be truthful, I hadn't even thought of it'. When we discussed it further, she said that DNA was 'just blood', and again that 'there's nothing about a blood sample that would frighten me whereas it might if people didn't know anything about it'.

Mr Watson, on the other hand, clearly had little idea what was involved in terms of the detail of the study. This was underlined when he asked me when he could expect to hear about the results of the blood tests. He commented that although he had been given information on the study, he hadn't 'had a chance to read all the bumph'. When asked about his views on the use of the DNA for analysis he said that 'up until you'd mentioned it I hadn't given it a second thought', but when we discussed this further he didn't see the analysis of (his) DNA as a problem. A third example is that of Mrs Reece. When I asked her to describe the study to me 'as if I were a friend or somebody who doesn't know anything about it', her description of the study bore a close resemblance to my understanding of it in general terms, but did not include a reference to the genetic analysis. The main attraction of participating in this particular study for her (and others) was that it did not involve taking unknown drugs. When I asked her about DNA, she said: 'I don't think I've really thought about it'.

Individuals may consent or refuse fairly unknowingly to a study. Thus framing the analysis in terms of a dichotomy between consent and non-consent may obscure some underlying dynamics of participation (see Haimes and Whong-Barr this volume). In this research study as in many others, respondents may formally be on record as having 'consented' because a signature is in place on a consent form, whilst not actively wishing to participate or having some reservations. Furthermore their position on participation in a research project may well change over time. In this case, all but one of the interviewees indicated that the use of DNA was not seen as a particular issue, rather it was often seen to be like most other blood tests. Even where they had not been aware that DNA analysis was a part of the study (and one to which they had consented in writing) they nevertheless expressed a willingness to hand over a small blood sample for this kind of testing. One man who found my questions particularly difficult said to me after the interview that the blood was 'entrusted', and should be used as the researchers saw fit. I took this as indicating both that he felt he had very limited expertise to judge or comment on the details of the research, and that he had chosen to trust the researchers. Many felt that genetic research was now very much on the agenda and could be seen as an indicator of good modern science, and so in a sense was not particularly novel, troubling or noteworthy.

'Everybody has their own DNA'

Many discussions about involvement in genetic research stress the 'need to know' about genetic tests, and a sense of 'genetic responsibility' on the part of participants in relation to family members (Hallowell 1999, Human Genetics Commission 2001) or even 'genetic solidarity' (Human Genetics Commission 2002). This emphasis was not so prominent in these interviews, as one might expect, given the nature of the disease: psoriatic arthritis is generally considered to have a complex multifactorial aetiology, although the unit is investigating a possible genetic component of the disease. (The condition has not to date been considered primarily a genetic disease.) Thus the rationale for the genetic study can fit with the multilayered models of illness which people often deploy.

Most respondents in this study insisted that the use of DNA in this context is not particularly 'special'. A brief extract from my interview with one of the respondents, Mrs Collier, is included here to illustrate this perspective. ('I' stands for interviewer and 'R' for the respondent, Mrs Collier.)

I: Now with the analysis of this genetic material, the DNA you know some people have concerns about DNA because [. . .] it's unique, my DNA is unique to me and yours to you . . .

R: My body, your body.

I: Yes and you know some people feel they've got worries about privacy or you know that kind of thing, do you have any sort of concerns on that score?

R: No because I am who I am, I've got nothing to hide, I've got nothing to show. I'm just a normal working person that's trying to get through life you know some days are good some days are bad. No because there's nothing in me that, you know it's the same as a toe nail or the same as a hand nail, the same as a bit of skin it's just me.

I: Right.

R: It's nothing special and if they can use it . . .

I: You see some people think it is some people think it's . . .

R: Privacy is your bank account because you know how much you're in the red (laughs).

I: Now that's critical.

R: Exactly, exactly, privacy is the way you run your life, not the way your life is, what you're made of is it really? You can't change the way you are made. You can change the way you run your life, you can change the way you are in life you can change the way you are as a person but you can't change the bits inside no matter how, I mean if it's inside me it's still me.

Towards the end of this extract we see the understanding that DNA *is* special in the sense that it is seen as an intrinsic part of (one)self. But in being part of the self, like a hand or toe nail, it is not seen as particularly vulnerable or sacred. Therefore its manipulation in legitimate medical research was not seen to be a particular concern. For many, the photographs of the skin condition which were taken by the research nurse were seen to be more worrying or invasive than the use of the blood sample for analysis of the DNA. For this group of interviewed research participants, then, DNA itself was not accorded a special status in relation to the need for protection of integrity or privacy. As one respondent said when probed on this question: 'it's just blood. At the end of

the day if it's something to do with your genes they need to look at it now
. . . I don't really understand. I marvel that they can do so much and find out
so much'.

However, DNA was seen to be special in another sense: the potential
of genetic techniques to lead to breakthroughs in research. These interviews
underlined how involvement in a genetic study can be intertwined with a
sense of hope and with the expectation of a more specific outcome than is
expected by the research team. The 'political economy of hope' in relation to
involvement in genetic research has been addressed by a number of authors
(see Stockdale 1999, Novas 2001). Such expectations also underline the way
in which research volunteers, whilst deploying substantial knowledge and
resources, also grapple with the limitations of their knowledge and expertise.
The stress within the sociological literature on lay knowledge has tended
to obscure the important implications of such limitations for the relations of
research participation.

From within this case study it is possible to sketch out participants'
approaches to participation in the genetic research in the context of their
relationship to the medical system more generally. Some respondents described
the development of their relationship with their doctors to one where their
own expertise is recognized: this group includes many who have no technical
or related expertise to draw on. A second group described how they were able
to deploy their knowledge of and access to the scientific literature to make
a judgement about the research. And third, some interviewees described their
own stance as one of trusting the doctor '100 per cent', and contrasted this
stance with that of others who 'read up'. Despite the diversity of approaches
taken to medical information and the medical system in general though, a
similar approach was taken to my questions about DNA by each of the three
respondents cited above. In their responses to my questions on possible
concerns about the use of genetic techniques, each stressed the importance of
these being deployed to investigate cause: Mrs Collier again:

> Well nowadays I mean you hear more and more about the genetic side of
> things, it's only like in the last ten years that they've started looking into
> you know the hereditary side of things. And I think a lot of it is linked
> an awful lot. And if they can find a genetic link in between, I mean like
> you say it could only be one tiny little chromosome, one tiny little thing
> that could link thousands of people together. I mean it's only when you
> actually look inside your body and you see what it's actually made of that
> it's a bit like scary. So I mean as far as I'm concerned if they can find
> something from that side of things then, I believe in what they're doing
> I believe that there is . . .

The place of the university and the NHS as research hosts was critical to
such confidence. This point was rarely made explicitly, but emerged from

responses to the contrasting question: 'if you had been approached by a commercial company undertaking the same kind of research (and entailing the same kind of contribution), would you have taken a different view?' In response most said specifically that they would take a different view, would not participate, although a few expressed a more balanced perspective on this. The institutional frameworks for the genetic research are clearly critical for this group. This echoes other research, in which doctors, and scientists in the university sector, are accorded a higher level of confidence than scientists working in industry.[6] Returning to those interviewed as part of my own research, the dimensions and shape of confidence in the research varied within these groups. For some, the trust expressed reflected an explicit weighing up of the possibility of risk, and finding it to be low.[7] For others, the confidence expressed conveyed rather a sense of faith. For most, the familiarity of the NHS and its allied institutions (including the university) seemed to be an important underlying condition.

Conclusion

The qualitative study discussed in this chapter was not designed to gather 'attitudes' from representatives of the general population.[8] Rather it aimed to draw on the reflections of those interviewed in conjunction with my own observations to unpack assumptions about participation in (epidemiological) genetic research. We have seen how, in the majority of interviews, DNA was not seen as 'special' in itself. No case is made here for research using genetic techniques to be seen as exceptional: the questions discussed here apply more generally to the contemporary phenomenon of involvement in research and more specifically to blood donation in that context. However, the scale of UK Biobank, which aims to be the largest such collection in the world, and the range of data to be collected[9] do constitute a new departure in organizing research. These developments can be seen as part of a trend of 'socialization of medical innovation' in that such innovations now demand the active participation of a wide range of lay people as participants (Webster 2002: 448).

Beginning with a consideration of the sociological literature, a number of points have been made about the dynamics of knowledge and trust. We have seen how the limitations of the knowledge which donors had were allied with a choice to place trust in the organizational host of the research. In the case studies referred to here, it appears that the familiarity of the university and the NHS facilitated trust in the research. There is little work on the cultural dimensions of such trust. In the case of the NHS, such work might usefully explore the way in which trust in these institutions has been buttressed by medical paternalism and patient deference. Further study of the ways in which trust is invested in specific social domains such as these would contribute a counterpoint to the overarching presence of grand(ish) theories about trust in much of the sociological literature. Finally, some further consideration of the dynamics of knowledge in research participation is due. Deflected by the analytical and political emphasis on lay expertise, the implications of the limitations of our expertise in relation to more complex (new) technologies have not received a great deal of attention in the recent sociological literature.

These points can inform our review of the principles which conventionally inform bioethics. The limitations that we have seen in relying on the ideal of informed consent go beyond the operational problems of putting such an ideal into practice: they are bound up with issues about asymmetries of knowledge and information. These are particularly acute in the case of blood donation for genetic research, where some of the responsibility for judging research is implicitly passed on to those who may not be well placed to do so.

The critique to which this chapter aims to contribute goes further than a questioning of concepts like informed consent. It is a more general challenge to the way that the policies, discourses and institutions of bioethics have often seemed to float above the specificity of the lives, circumstances and histories of individuals and communities. This can be related to the importance of universality and foundationalism for (modernist) philosophers as they have sought to 'compose and impose an all-important unitary ethics' (Bauman 1993: 6; Haimes 2002). This is perhaps what divides authors in this field who agree on much else. For some of us, however much we might agree with the principles of the bioethics rubric, the deployment of reified principles to deal with a complex social question is problematic. An example here is the call by Chadwick and Berg for a shift towards 'solidarity and equity' (2001: 320) as a framework for considering genetic research. Such ideals are admirable and indeed influential, but I suggest that the imposition of a new rubric takes us no further in addressing the problems entailed in participation in large-scale biobanks. As Arthur Kleinman noted, with reference to another idealized concept deployed in discussions of the ethics of research participation, different interests will be at play in relation to such projects:

> Beneficent social contracts make good philosophical theory, but they deny empirical evidence in local social worlds . . . real communities are sources of suffering at least as much as of assistance. They do not contain explicit social contracts, but they are filled with different interests, status divisions, class divisions, ethnic conflicts, and factionalism.
>
> (Kleinman, 1995: 48)

A similar issue arises with the ideal of 'gift relationships'. Reviewing the seminal idea of blood donation as a 'gift' in the light of my discussions with contemporary blood donors, I was struck by the emphasis on a very practical kind of reciprocity. Donors talked of making provision for the supply of blood which may be needed by family, friends and strangers at any time. Such an interpretation of reciprocity is of course specific to the nature of blood donation in the UK, where there is a long history allied with the welfare system as a whole, and the technologies involved are widely acceptable. To some extent the ideal of practical reciprocity combined with a loyalty to the NHS is echoed in the discussions with donors of blood for the genetic research project. However, the relationship between that ideal of reciprocity and the way that genetic research is organized is less clear: the benefits from blood donation for research are less tangible. We know less about how that research is organized, what benefits will emerge and how they will be distributed.

It is interesting that the practicalities of such reciprocity seem not to permeate the policy discussions about genetic databanks. Thus we hear little about the small but tangible benefits which may be important to blood donors and research participants. These may include the perceived advantages of being cared for and 'checked out' within a screening process for blood donation. A number of respondents in focus groups conducted as part of a consultation commissioned by the UK Biobank funding partners, the MRC and the Wellcome Trust, raised the issue of health checks for participants (People, Science and Policy 2002: 16). However this appears not to have been taken at face value as an expectation of practical reciprocity to be addressed by the biobank organizers. Rather this is deemed to be a problem of information, with a recommendation that the lack or limitations of such checks be made clear to participants (People, Science and Policy 2002: 17). Respondents also raised the issue of the potential for pharmaceutical companies to profit from the use of their donations (People, Science and Policy 2002: 20–21). This possibility is widely acknowledged but unresolved. Whereas some recent policy papers endeavour to harness the ideal of (patient) altruism to a rhetoric of progress and prosperity,[10] these matters could perhaps usefully be considered within a framework of practical reciprocity.

A broader implication emerges from the emphasis blood donors place on making shared provision for risks.[11] The emphasis on shared risks refers us back to the concerns which led Titmuss to undertake his comparative study on blood donation. Whilst the ideal of the 'gift relationship' recurs like a leitmotif throughout several decades of subsequent discussion on blood donation, Titmuss' underlying concerns with 'the ways in which society organizes and structures . . . its health and welfare systems' (Titmuss 1997: 292) are rarely addressed in these discussions. His substantive work was about such systems, and the implications he thought the structures we devise for them had for social integration or alienation. Those charged with organizing large databases of genetic information such as UK Biobank are likely to find it useful to address the more structural questions: who benefits and in what ways from (blood) donations and what is the appropriate place for commerce in this new research endeavour? Adopting a language of altruism will not in itself resolve these issues.

Acknowledgements

The qualitative study discussed in this paper was funded through a training grant from the Wellcome Trust. I would like to thank Paul Martin and Robert Dingwall at the University of Nottingham for their support and supervision of this work, Alison Taylor for transcribing interviews and Mike Sandys for his help. I would also like to acknowledge the kind assistance of those within the host organizations who facilitated access for research interviews. Conclusions drawn are my own as are any errors.

Notes

1. See Kaye and Martin's (2000) discussion 'Safeguards for research using large-scale DNA collections' for an overview of some of the implications of these developments.
2. See for example People, House of Lords (2001), Human Genetics Commission (2002), and Science and Policy (2002).
3. As is well known, Titmuss' concept of 'gift relationship' was influenced by his reading of first and second generations of anthropologists – who wrote before the development of blood transfusion services. The ideal of reciprocity has been an overarching norm in anthropology (Weiner 1992). The more empirical and particular turn of ethnography in recent years though, undermines the fixing of gift giving into one set of meanings. An important contribution to the contemporary literature on gift relationships was triggered by Bourdieu's examination of the pattern of gift exchanges over time (Bourdieu 1977). Bourdieu emphasized the way in which gift giving constructed social bonds and obligations as burdensome as those of economic debt. Ultimately, the ideology of apparently disinterested gift giving is seen as being no more and no less than an imposition of – and complicity with – a symbolic meaning.
4. See Webster (2002) for a review of these approaches in this context.
5. That is, a disease with a clear cut genetic aetiology such as the rare disorders caused by mutations in single genes.
6. See for example the report on 'Europeans and Biotechnology in 2002' (Gaskell et al. 2003).
7. A useful distinction can be made between trust 'which allows for risk-taking decisions' and confidence which does not involve a consideration of alternatives (Luhman 2000: 4).
8. The funding bodies have commissioned several large studies to gather data of this kind from stratified samples of the UK population. These include People Science and Policy Limited (2002), and The Wellcome Trust and MRC (2000).
9. Only some of that data are genetic data, and a number of my respondents considered that other personal data may be more sensitive.
10. See the report from House of Lords Select Committee (2001) Report on Human Genetic Databases for one such example.
11. This is reminiscent of a point made by Lupton and Tulloch in their discussion of interviews with Australians about their perceptions of risk: here they point to a sense of risk as being shared, 'spread over more than one body/self'. This they

suggest, 'represents an aspect of risk identity that is little recognized in the major tenets of the risk identity thesis, with their emphasis on the atomized, risk avoiding individual' (Lupton and Tulloch 2002: 324).

References

Apthorpe, R. (1997). 'Policy as language and power', in C. Shore and S. Wright (eds) *Anthropology of Policy: Critical Perspectives on Governance and Power*, London: Routledge.

Bauman, Z. (1993). *Postmodern Ethics*, Oxford: Blackwell.

Beck, U. (1992). *Risk Society: Towards a New Modernity*, London: Sage.

Berger, A. (2001). 'UK genetics database plans revealed', *British Medical Journal* 322: 1018.

Bourdieu, P. (1977). *Outline of a Theory of Practice (Cambridge Studies in Social Anthropology, 16)*, trans. Richard Nice, Cambridge: Cambridge University Press.

Chadwick, R. and Berg, K. (2001). 'Solidarity and equity: new ethical frameworks for genetic databases', *Nature* 318: 318–321.

Collins, H. and Evans, R. (2002). 'The third wave of science studies: studies of expertise and experience', *Social Studies of Science* 33: 235–296.

Davison, C., Davey Smith, G. and Frankel, S. (1991). 'Lay epidemiology and the prevention paradox: the implications of coronary candidacy for health education', *Sociology of Health and Illness* 13: 1–20.

Dingwall, R. (2002). 'Bioethics', in A. Pilnick (ed.) *Genetics and Society: An Introduction*, Buckingham: Open University Press, pp. 161–180.

Edwards, J. (1999). 'Expertise in understandings of new reproductive and genetic technologies', in Public Understanding of Science Newsletter, ESRC New Opportunities Programme in PUS, 7: British Library.

Elliott, A. (2002). 'Beck's sociology of risk: a critical assessment', *Sociology* 35: 293–315.

Fox, R. and Swazey, J. (1992). *Spare Parts*, Oxford: Oxford University Press.

Frank, A. (2000). 'Social bioethics and the critique of autonomy: review essay', *Health* 4: 378–394.

Gaskell, G., Allum, N., Stares, S. *et al.* (2003). *Europeans and Biotechnology in 2002: Eurobarometer 58.0* (2nd edn): A report to the EC Directorate General for Research from the Project 'Life Sciences in European Society' QLG7-CT-1999-00286.

Giddens, A. (1990). *The Consequences of Modernity*, Oxford: Polity Press.

Haimes, E. (2002). 'What can the social sciences contribute to the study of ethics? Theoretical, empirical and substantive contributions', *Bioethics* 16: 89–113.

Hallowell, N. (1999). 'Doing the right thing: genetic risk and responsibility', in P. Conrad and J. Gabe (eds) *Sociological Perspectives on the New Genetics*, Oxford: Blackwell.

House of Lords Select Committee on Science and Technology (2001). Human genetic databases: challenges and opportunities, House of Lords, Session 2000–01, 4th report, London: Stationery Office.

Human Genetics Commission (2001). 'Whose hands on your genes?' A discussion document on the storage protection and use of personal information, London: Department of Health.

Human Genetics Commission (2002). Inside information: balancing interests in the use of personal genetic data. Available HTTP: <www.hgc.gov.uk/inside information> (accessed February 2003).

Kaye, J. and Martin, P. (2000). 'Safeguards for research using large scale DNA collections', *British Medical Journal* 321: 1146–1149.

Kleinman, A. (1995). *Writing at the Margin: Discourse between Anthropology and Medicine*, Berkeley: University of California Press.

Luhman, N. (2000). 'Familiarity, confidence, trust: problems and alternatives', in D. Gambetta (ed.) *Trust: Making and Breaking Cooperative Relations*, electronic edition. Online. Available HTTP: <http://www.sociology.ox.ac/papers/luhman94–107.doc> (accessed on 12 May 2003).

Lupton, D. and Tulloch, J. (2002). '"Risk is part of your life": risk epistemologies amongst a group of Australians', *Sociology* 36: 317–334.

Medical Research Council (2001). *Human Tissue and Biological Samples for Use in Research: Operational and Ethical Guidelines*, London: MRC Ethics Series.

Novas, C. (2001). 'The political economy of hope: the labour of expecting cures'. Paper presented at *Postgraduate Forum on Genetics and Society Conference*, University of Nottingham, June 2001.

O'Neill, O. (2002). *Autonomy and Trust in Bioethics*, Cambridge: Cambridge University Press.

People, Science and Policy Ltd (2002). Biobank UK: A question of trust: a consultation. Report prepared for the Medical Research Council and the Wellcome Trust.

Piliavin, J. (1990). 'Why do they give the gift of life? A review of research on blood donors since 1977', *Transfusion* 30: 444–459.

Robinson, E. and Murray, A. (1999). 'Altruism: is it alive and well? Proceedings of the international seminar, Royal College of Pathologists, 13 November 1998', *Transfusion Medicine* 9: 351–382.

Simmons, R.G., Marine Klein, S. and Simmons, R.L. (1987). *Gift of Life: The Effect of Organ Transplantation on Individual, Family and Social Dynamics*, Oxford: Transaction Books.

Stapleton, H., Kirkham, M. and Thomas, G. (2002). 'Qualitative study of evidence based leaflets in maternity care', *British Medical Journal* 324: 639.

Stockdale, A. (1999). 'Waiting for the cure: mapping the social relations of human gene therapy research', in P. Conrad and J. Gabe (eds) *Sociological Perspectives on the New Genetics*, *Sociology of Health and Illness monograph series*, Oxford: Blackwell.

Titmuss, R. (1997). *The Gift Relationship: From Human Blood to Social Policy*, in A. Oakley and J. Ashton (eds) (original edition with new chapters), London: LSE Books.

Tutton, R. (2002). 'Gift relationships in genetic research', *Science as Culture* 11(4): 523–542.

Webster, A. (2002). 'Innovative health technologies and the social: redefining health, medicine and the body', *Current Sociology* 50: 443–457.

Weiner, A. (1992). *Inalienable Possessions: The Paradox of Keeping-while-Giving*, Berkeley: University of California Press.

Wellcome Trust and Medical Research Council (2000). *Public Perceptions of Human Biological Samples*, London: Wellcome Trust.

Williams, G. and Popay, J. (1994). 'Lay knowledge and the privilege of experience', in J. Gabe, D. Kelleher and G. Williams (eds) *Challenging Medicine*, London: Routledge.

Wynne, B. (1991). 'Knowledges in context', *Science, Technology and Human Values* 16: 111–121.

Chapter 4

Levels and styles of participation in genetic databases

A case study of the North Cumbria Community Genetics Project

Erica Haimes and Michael Whong-Barr

Introduction

This chapter draws upon data generated by a Wellcome Trust-funded study of the North Cumbria Community Genetics Project (NCCGP), one of the longest standing genetic databases in the UK. One important strand in our research is broadly concerned with establishing how and why individuals decide to donate, or refuse to donate, samples and lifestyle information to a genetic database. As this formulation suggests, there is a tendency in much of the literature (see below) to refer to two categories of responses to the request to provide samples and information (agreement or refusal) and to the individuals as either donors or non-donors. However, the evidence from our study suggests that the responses are actually rather more nuanced than this and that this apparently simple distinction requires further exploration.

It is clear from the data that there are varying levels of donation and non-donation and that there are different ways in which individuals donate or do not donate to such a database. Therefore, rather than use the terms 'donation' or 'non-donation' as descriptors, which imply a single meaning attached to a simple, one-way act, we use the notion of 'participation' to begin to reflect what is in fact a highly varied social process, with multiple meanings. By examining the levels and styles of participation from a number of different perspectives we seek to capture the variations in the meanings and processes attached to the decision-making around this aspect of genetic databases. This then leads to a broader discussion of the context in which the request to donate to such a database lies and the associated issues raised by the responses to this request, at both individual and community levels.

The overall aim of our study was to investigate the perceptions of women in Cumbria, in the north-west of England, who have been asked to donate tissue samples and complete a health and lifestyle questionnaire for the NCCGP. In particular the study sought to compare and contrast the perceptions and attitudes of those who have agreed to donate to the NCCGP with those who have declined, to assess whether there are distinct differences between the two responses. This study will provide practical feedback to the NCCGP and will also contribute much needed data to inform the wider debates over the acceptability of genetic databases to potential donors.

Genetics research is increasingly looking for gene–disease associations. This requires large-scale biological sample collections, combined with personal medical information, to be used for epidemiological analysis. Whilst acknowledging the debates about definition (King 2000) we shall refer to such collections of information as 'genetic databases'. Normative frameworks on the ethics of genetic databases, as well as questions about their political and practical purpose and use, focus on issues such as informed consent, confidentiality, the use and possible misuse of samples and information, and questions about feedback to donors (House of Lords 2000, 2001, Human Genetics Commission 2000, 2002, Kaye and Martin 2000, Rose 2000, Spallone and Wilkie 2000, Voss 2000, Berger 2001, Beskow *et al.* 2001, Meade and Hopkinson 2001, Staley 2001, Hansard 2002, People, Science and Policy 2002, Wade 2002, Weisbrot 2003). Such issues are particularly pertinent given the proposal by the UK Medical Research Council and the Wellcome Trust to establish the UK BioBank national genetic database. A central question concerns the acceptability of databases to the public (Lowrance 2001).

A study by Cragg Ross Dawson (2000) indicates that while 'the public' is initially willing to donate to such collections it is unaware of the full implications of so doing and when informed about the wider issues respondents then became concerned about the reliability of safeguards to protect confidentiality, the possible misuse of their personal information by researchers, employers, insurance companies, police, pharmaceutical and commercial enterprises, the rights of donors to receive feedback on their samples, and whether consent could be truly informed when the future use of samples remains uncertain. This study reveals that many of these concerns relate to how much trust the public has in the medical profession and the government (these issues have been raised by others too; see for example, House of Lords 2000, Kaye and Martin 2000, Spallone and Wilkie 2000). Finally, following further discussion with respondents, Cragg Ross Dawson's study discovered that exploring these concerns led to respondents feeling better informed and more positive about donation again.

These, briefly, are the views of general members of 'the public'. However, we know little about the views of those who have actually been asked to donate to a genetic database (but see also EPEG Project 2001). We need to know the views and values of such people and, in particular, their reasons for either agreeing, or refusing, to assist future discussions on the ethical implications of genetic databases and to assist policy-making in this area. Such data would also clarify the wider sociocultural significance of such databases. The need for these data has been described as a 'fundamental issue' (Spallone and Wilkie 2000). The NCCGP provided a rare opportunity to study such a population.

The North Cumbria Community Genetics Project

The NCCGP aims to assist the identification of gene–disease associations, and the impact of environmental factors on those associations. They do this by providing a large-scale source of DNA, plasma and viable cells from a normal population, linked to information about lifestyle, that can then be subjected to genetic epidemiological analysis. Blood and tissue samples are collected from the umbilical cord of newborn babies and information about health and lifestyles is collected via brief questionnaires completed by mothers. So far NCCGP data have been used in projects on heart disease, cancer and neural tube defects. An ethics advisory group advises the NCCGP on procedures and the use of samples (Chase *et al.* 1998).

The NCCGP raises similar social and ethical issues to those already mentioned. It could also be argued that it raises some social and ethical issues specific to its own procedures. The latter might include: first, requesting samples from a 'captive audience' of women (Garcia 1990, Jacobus 1990) receiving antenatal care (albeit with the assurance that refusal does not compromise treatment); second, requesting mothers to give consent on behalf of their babies (the child can withdraw their sample at the age of 16) (Clarke 1998, Mason and McCall Smith 1999); and third, requesting mothers to give named lifestyle information about their partners. Finally, British Nuclear Fuels Limited (BNFL) were involved in the initial funding of the NCCGP. BNFL have a major base in Cumbria at Sellafield which has been associated with allegations about the effects of excessive radiation causing a higher than average incidence of childhood leukaemia.

None the less, the NCCGP claims a high response rate. By 2002, over seven thousand samples had been collected. This means that nearly 90 per cent of the pregnant women approached agree to provide umbilical cord samples and, since 1999, maternal blood specimens (Chase *et al.* 2000). In light of the Cragg Ross Dawson study this response rate raises some questions. Is it the case that participants in the NCCGP: (a) are well disposed towards the NCCGP and are not fully aware of the implications of donating samples and information, or (b) do not have the same concerns as those expressed elsewhere, or (c) perceive the benefits of the NCCGP to outweigh any concerns, or (d) feel their concerns have been fully addressed by the NCCGP team and their anxieties allayed, or (e) have a range of other views, interests and concerns that have not yet come to light?

A small minority of the women approached did not participate in the NCCGP. Initial discussions with the NCCGP team suggested that this could be because some women are missed out by mistake or some make a conscious decision not to participate. Possible reasons for refusal were thought to include concerns similar to those already cited (and a view that the NCCGP failed to address them sufficiently) or an organized opposition to the NCCGP because of the involvement of BNFL (Chase *et al.* 1998).

Studying the 'black box' of participation

The extent to which 'donation' and 'non-donation' are attributable to primarily local factors such as BNFL, or to other, more widely held, interests and concerns, and the extent to which 'non-donation' represents a distinct stance to that of 'donation', are matters for empirical investigation. Such an investigation opens up the 'black box' of the social processes of decision-making, that lie between the request to donate and the collection of samples and information. This box needs to be opened since the NCCGP could be cited as a model to be duplicated elsewhere, for example in the UK Biobank and even internationally as it appears to work in practical terms. If this is the case, it is necessary to identify, from the potential donors' point of view, which aspects are the most persuasive and to ensure that they are capable of duplication elsewhere.

Equally though, it could be argued that the apparent success of NCCGP is based on misunderstandings by the 'donors' of what it is they are agreeing to, in which case the practical benefits are achieved at social and ethical costs. Perhaps 'non-donors' are better informed about the implications as it has been suggested that those who are most informed about bioscience have the most polarized views (Voss 2000). Also, only 60 per cent of those approached complete the 'mother's questionnaire' (a health and lifestyle questionnaire for the woman and her partner) as well as donating samples. The reasons for this 'partial donation' need examining to see whether 'donors' distinguish between the two types of information and, if so, how and why (Martin 2000).

All these possibilities need to be considered and need to be informed by data that reveal the knowledge, values and processes of donors' and non-donors' decision-making (Spallone and Wilkie 2000). Also, because of this variation, it is clear that the notion of 'donation', with its implications, at least in the ways in which it is used in the policy-making and clinical literature already cited, of a relatively simple one-way act of giving something to someone else, is inadequate. A phrase such as 'participation', which implies a more active process of engagement with, and sharing in the creation of, the database, is more useful. It acknowledges that those who are approached to give samples and information have an active role in creating the database, including those who decline to provide these items since that too shapes the database achieved and there are degrees of involvement and variations in the style of that involvement.

We conducted 50 interviews with potential donors, 43 of whom would conventionally be labelled as 'participants' and 7 as 'non-participants' (although, as we shall see, this is an inadequate distinction). We had foreseen problems recruiting non-participants and so used a wide range of strategies, such as articles and adverts in local newspapers, snowball sampling from other non-participants and community opposition groups, presentations to mother and toddler groups, to increase their number with limited success. Our two key research questions were: What is the repertoire of perceptions, concerns, views and understandings that women raise as part of the process of deciding whether to participate or not? And are there differences in perceptions, concerns, views and understandings, or in the importance attached to these, between those who identify as participants and those who identify as non-participants?

As well as interviewing those who had been asked to donate samples we also interviewed members of the NCCGP research team and members of the opposition groups. We speculated that these two additional sets of interviews would yield a range of competing normative statements as to why women should or should not donate samples to the NCCGP (Haimes and Whong-Barr 2003).

Levels of participation

From a technical point of view, in terms of the design of the NCCGP as a database, 'full participation' would mean that a woman contributed umbilical cord samples from her baby, a blood sample from herself and health and life-style information about herself and her partner by completing a document known as the 'mother's questionnaire'. 'Partial participation' would mean a donation of the cord samples and blood but no lifestyle information. 'Non-participation' would mean that nothing was given to the database at all. However, during our interviews with the various groups, these apparently clear distinctions became increasingly blurred as interviewees sought to explain how and why potential participants made their decisions over donation. In addition, there were variations in the significance attributed to the differing levels of participation.

Interviews with the NCCGP research team indicate a relaxed attitude to the actual participation rates they have achieved, especially as these were frequently referred to as being between 80 and 90 per cent, even though this is actually the figure for 'partial participation' rather than 'full participation'. Comments from the interviews with the NCCGP team minimized the involvement needed from donors; one said that they assumed that the donations were 'given and forgotten about' and that they would not want women to be worried about the donation, nor did the team wish to 'lean on them' to donate (T234). The idea was to make potential donors 'comfortable to say no' (T587) and that if there had been a 100 per cent participation rate the team would be worried that they were overselling the project (T351).

One referred to the 'huge body of altruism in the general public' as an explanation for such a high response rate, which was not seen as a surprise (T587). Another suggested that 'people on average do have an altruistic streak and mostly people are happy to be involved in medical research that they can see might be of greater good' (T081). Another important element was the trust that most people had in the National Health Service and in its professionals

(T234), as well as in the fact that the data were being processed by a local research institute and a local reputable university (T351). However, an over-whelming reason for the high participation was, according to one member, the fact that: 'We are just taking samples that are normally thrown away and I feel that's a very strong reason why the NCCGP is so successful' (T351). This was echoed by all the other members of the team as well: 'I think most people feel reasonably optimistic that it doesn't impact on them particu-larly and all they are doing is giving samples that would otherwise not be used' (T177); 'there is nothing to lose' (T587); 'we are not asking much, people don't have to do very much to be part of it, it doesn't take up their time' (T081).

This last set of quotes shows very clearly that 'participation' in the minds of the NCCGP team has come to mean, primarily, giving the blood and tissue samples. The mother's questionnaire is a document printed on purple paper, with questions on 12 sides of A5, covering the woman's and her partner's sociodemographic profiles, their own health, their history of smoking, their employment history and their family histories of long-term or serious illness. Explanations for partial participation (that is, the non-completion of this questionnaire) were mixed. One suggested:

> That is apathy, definitely. If they don't have time to do it when you are seeing them, quite often things are always in a rush, if you try to make them make a start on it, I think they would then fill it in. I think if they don't start it, they just can't be bothered. Other than that, people do not like to give information, it does ask for addresses, where you have lived for the last 5 years, a bit about your education. I think a few ladies do feel that it is not necessary to have all that information for the research, you could just have a postcode or perhaps it could be a bit more anonymous.
>
> (T033)

Another drew an interesting distinction between the types of donation:

> I'm not surprised that people are reluctant to give personal details, because a sample is a sample, stick a number on a sample and it doesn't give any information, there's nothing personal about it almost. It's giving biochemical genetic information that will be useful for disease studies research but it doesn't given any personal details. You know, there is nothing associated with it that can be linked to the person as it were. The questionnaire, yes, I'm not altogether surprised that people are reluctant to fill it in. As you probably know more women fill it in than their partners so they have a lot of what we jokingly say is immaculate conceptions, you know, got the details on the mother but not the father . . . A minor or smaller factor is probably the fact that there is higher illiteracy in West

Cumbria. Now if people don't wish to admit to being illiterate they might not wish to fill in a questionnaire.

(T351)

Thus the type of information being asked for and the context in which it was being requested (during pregnancy) was seen as an inhibiting factor:

> Like all questionnaires, people prefer not to fill them in, there are very few people who love filling in questionnaires . . . and the smoking issue is something that is interesting . . . they know they shouldn't be smoking, but people don't like actually having to admit to it either, I suspect there is an element of that too. I don't know, I have not seen it as my role to actually ask too much of participants what they feel about the questionnaire because I've . . . taken a hands off line there. I have offered it to them and let it at that really.

(T587)

The extent to which this partial participation was seen to 'matter' also varied amongst the research team. One view was 'I think it does matter' (T033); another was uncertain:

> How it affects the project, I don't know because I don't think we have had a collaborative study so far that has used any data from the mother's questionnaire at all . . . So I think that you'll probably find that although it was about 60 per cent to start with that filled in all or part of the questionnaire, I believe it's dropped a bit now, since then. As I say, I can understand that but I don't know what impact that will have on the project as a whole.

(T351)

This lack of demand from other researchers wanting to use the mother's questionnaire data perhaps explains the team's relaxed attitude to this aspect of their study:

> Most of the information that has been sent out has been anonymous with no attached data so the questionnaire information hasn't been required. It would be nice to have full ascertainment, it would be wonderful, but I mean we can still function as a facility . . .

(T469)

Similarly, another argued:

> It is obviously much better to have more complete data and it reduces the power of your study if you have missing data . . . but the compliance rate

is pretty high . . . it's a very short questionnaire and it captures the minimum amount of information and any really in-depth study using health information would need to look at other sources.

(T081)

The team also minimized the reasons for non-participation. One reason was that such women were 'lost in the system', another that most people who do not donate simply forget, 'there's nothing systematic about it' (T081). The views were summed up by one member who said the 15 per cent non-participation was a 'grey area' which they could not be clear about, but on the other hand, another team member was keen to point out again that the team do not ask people why they refuse, as this was 'not suitable' (T587).

Whilst interviewees from the community opposition groups had little to say about the different types of donation elicited or the different levels of participation, they shared similar views to the research team about the reasons for the high participation rate, though they saw reasons to be concerned about this:

I would assume that it's that high partly for the reason that we've already said. People are assured that what they are doing is being done in absolute total confidence and the other part is, 'well, this is BNFL and BNFL are not going to mislead us and Newcastle [University], why should they mislead us about anything?' People are not going to question the motives about this if it's put to them in a straightforward way, 'this is really useful information, we can build on this, use it in all kinds of helpful ways', people are not going to say no to it. In a way, maybe I feel that people are being taken advantage of, that maybe the whole thing isn't explained as fully as it should be. Maybe if [one of us] was included on a counselling team and was able to put another perspective of this project to the potential donor, then maybe it would be different.

(C002)

As we shall discuss further in the following section, this comment is tied to a view about why those who chose to donate to the NCCGP made this decision, a view, which, like those of the NCCGP team, is linked to ideas about styles of participation too. On the whole, those who apparently opposed the NCCGP were reluctant to make strong statements about the issues surrounding participation and why women ought not to participate. They were more outspoken about their opposition to the involvement of BNFL rather than to the NCCGP specifically. One acknowledged why some women might want to be part of this research:

Because I think, well, we all want some research, don't we? We all want to see that people are healthy. Particularly when you get emotive words like child cancer and spina bifida and all these other horrible diseases, neurone diseases. People say that they are doing research into cot deaths [a reference to a newspaper report in the early days of NCCGP when this was mentioned as a possible benefit to the research]. Of course we all want to be a part of that and if you think you can help, that's great.

(C001)

This wish to help is clearly expressed in the mothers' interviews, though interestingly it is expressed equally strongly by 'participants' as by 'non-participants'.

Whilst the NCCGP research team is not as concerned as might be expected about the differing levels of participation, although not as concerned as might be expected, the women, perhaps surprisingly, were very uncertain about the range of donations they were asked to give and just as unclear about what they did actually give. That is to say, most women who were interviewed as participants in the NCCGP were themselves not clear about whether they had in fact given all the samples and information that would constitute full participation. This is partly attributable to not remembering what they had been asked to give and partly to not being able to distinguish between the information and blood samples they were asked to give as part of routine antenatal care and that asked specifically for the NCCGP.

Difficulty in remembering what they had been asked to give was a recurring theme. In terms of the 'mother's questionnaire', despite its purple colour, many women said they did not remember ever seeing it, let alone completing it: 'No, I can't remember seeing one of those' (M007); 'I don't think so . . . certainly don't remember any purple paper (laughs)' (M070); 'No, I didn't fill out the purple form' (M046). Even those who thought they had completed it were vague about its contents and purpose. For example, 'I can't remember to be honest, I think I did. Is it all about me having a history, yes, I think I did' (M011); 'I wouldn't say I was totally clear on it, I can't remember, I just assumed, obviously, that they can relate it to medical [matters]' (M030). Similarly, with the maternal blood samples, there was a high level of uncertainty as to whether they were asked to provide one for the NCCGP, let alone whether they consented to doing so: 'No, I don't think so, I don't think I was asked to' (M002); 'I honestly don't know' (M044); 'I've no idea if they took one or not' (M049); 'If they'd wanted one I would have, but I can't remember' (M0101); 'No, I just think it was from the umbilical cord' (M046).

The difficulty many women had distinguishing between that which they were asked to provide for routine antenatal care and that asked for the NCCGP database applied to both the 'mother's questionnaire' and to the maternal blood samples. One woman said about the questionnaire:

Well, it's difficult to say because I filled that in at the same time as I filled in my medical notes . . . I had to fill that in as well and I think they were

both the same kind of questions . . . so I have trouble thinking which one
. . . I think maybe I did fill something in.

(M024)

Others said about the blood test:

I don't know whether I did or not . . . they're taking test tubes off you for
this, that and the other, it may well have been one of the other. I don't
know. I'm sorry I don't recall, no.

(M003)

No, I don't know . . . well, another test, one more to add to the list. You
know, the longer you're pregnant, the more things progress, the more tests
you have . . . '.

(M006)

and:

I'd imagine, yeah. I never refused anything that they asked me to do.

(M026)

Surprisingly there was even a small element of uncertainty amongst the
non-participants as to whether a maternal blood sample had been taken for the
NCCGP. One said that she had not given a sample, at least, 'not knowingly
. . . they took a lot of blood at my antenatal' (M060). Another said, 'They might
have taken one doing some of the antenatal stuff but I don't remember it. They
took so much blood that they could have' (M067). This is not meant to imply
that non-participants were suggesting that the NCCGP research team took
illicit samples from them. Rather, it simply indicates just how difficult it
is for any woman to be absolutely clear about who takes what samples, and for
what purposes, during antenatal care.

Both these elements, that of memory and that of distinguishing the prove-
nance of requests, could be explained in terms of their failings as individuals,
for example their poor memory and poor understanding perhaps because of
poor concentration. However, it would appear from the data, much more likely
to be attributable to the fact that they were asked for this information and
blood sample during pregnancy. Thus the social context of pregnancy raises
the ethical question of informed consent. If women are uncertain about what
they donated (and indeed most women were interviewed for our study within
weeks of giving birth, so memory attrition could not be attributed to passing
time alone), how clear can they be about the rationale of the research to which
they contributed, or about the nature of the uses to which their information
and samples would be put (see also O'Neill 2002 and Whong-Barr 2002)?
This brief point indicates just how important a notion of the level of participation is to a wiser understanding of participation in genetic databases.

Styles of participation

It is already apparent that a simple two-way distinction between women who decide to donate and women who decide not to donate does not reflect the complexities in the *levels* of participation, let alone in the reasons *why* some donate (even partially) and some do not. In trying to tease apart the reasons given in the interviews for 'participation' and 'refusal' it becomes clear that a core reason for donating (wishing to help) is rated as equally important by participants as by refusers. In addition, however, those who do donate expressed their wish to help in a number of different ways, which suggests that there are different *styles* to donating/helping.

Our analysis of the participating mothers' interviews reveals two very strong strands: a wish to help and the sense that not very much was involved in providing that help. The wish to help was expressed in a number of ways with different views as to who it was they wanted to help. Some felt their donation was helping the future in some unspecified way, others that it would help their own children's generation, others that it would help babies and children in general, or simply 'other people' in the future. A couple of women mentioned specifically helping Cumbria with their donations. This last point might be tied to another very common reason given for donating, which was to assist research into the eradication of disease:

> I would say it was just the sort of research for medical purposes, to help towards illnesses, such as cancer, Parkinsons, MS, all these types of things, yes, just to use them in connection with treatment in the future.
>
> (M012)

Several were aware that they themselves had benefited from research done previously and this influenced their own decisions:

> . . . because we had had the IVF treatment, you think, 'well, if they hadn't done a lot of research about that then', you know . . . I think that was the main reason why we agreed that we would donate. We thought that anything that helps, you know helps with cancer or anything like that. And there was no harm to me or the baby so we thought, well, 'yes, it's a good idea'.
>
> (M013)

> My understanding of what the Cumbria Genetics Project is about, it's something that is worth doing. My contribution to it is very small for me, it's not as if it was an ongoing thing, its not as if I'm being asked to do something every week or every year, it's a one off thing, it was a one off donation but really, you know it didn't impinge on me at all. I'm glad to have the opportunity to be involved in something like this because I think

it's important but it's not something that preys on my mind. I just think if you don't have medical research you don't move forward.

(M008)

This woman then went on to compare what was asked of her for the NCCGP with a project that her husband contributed to as a child when his mother agreed to have him be a 'guinea pig' for the measles vaccine.

. . . and at the end of the day what we did in giving a sample and afterbirth was nothing compared to actually having your child vaccinated with a vaccine that was, well it would have been through a lot of trials but was still, you know, at the forefront.

(M008)

This quotation is very useful in showing how these two strands intertwined. This sense that not a lot was involved was also expressed in a number of other ways. Interviews included remarks such as 'it was no harm to me or the baby'; 'there wasn't much involved'; 'it was no cost to me'; 'the afterbirth would just be thrown away otherwise'; 'it wasn't a big issue'; 'it was an easy decision to make'; 'there was no reason not to donate'; 'I don't know why I just did it'. For example:

It doesn't affect me personally, it's only part of the procedure which is gone anyway. I mean, after you have given birth, that is the last thing on your mind, I don't care what they do with it, they can do what they want with it. I don't need it anymore, the baby doesn't need it anymore, so you know it's matterless and they had to take blood anyway after you've had the baby so I mean it's just a little drop extra.

(M006)

' . . . it wasn't anything detrimental to me so if it helps somebody else in the future then they're more than welcome, particularly if I don't have to do the work' (M028). 'It's basically why not? I couldn't think of any good reason why not really' (M034).

Only one woman expressed regret at donating:

'Do you want to donate your umbilical cord?' I think someone said it was for asthma. Was it for asthma, I'm sure that what's somebody said it was for, something to do with asthma. And I don't know, at the time I said 'yes'. I wished I hadn't have done, I must admit. I really wished that I had more information and that I was better informed and I wish I wasn't put on the spot to make that decision because I don't think that I was in the right frame of mind to make the right decision.

(M040)

Participants (full and partial) speculate on why some women might refuse to donate. Most find it difficult to explain this but suggest that perhaps others are not like them:

> I just assumed why wouldn't anybody want to do it really but then again everybody is not like yourself so . . . I honestly couldn't think of any reason why women didn't do it, it's [the afterbirth] just to be taken away anyway, I don't know.
>
> (M030)

One respondent suggested that others perhaps needed to gain something themselves from donating: 'because most people are like that, aren't they? Most people if they are not getting anything back from it will not give, even if it is something they are not going to use' (M036). Thus helping is not just a worthwhile activity in its own right; the language of helping is also a way of establishing the sort of person that one is and of distancing oneself from the puzzling sort of person who does not want to help (see Haimes and Whong-Barr 2003).

Paradoxically, this use of the language of helping (Gustafsson-Stolt *et al.* 2002) is also present in the accounts of women who did not donate to the NCCGP. Those accounts indicate that these women are also keen to portray themselves as willing to help others, but just not in these particular circumstances. For instance one woman established the fact that she had donated stem cells to another project but was not happy to donate to the NCCGP because she thought the purpose of their research was vague and she also did not want to provide access to her medical records as she could not understand why this was needed. Another woman stressed how guilty she felt about not donating:

> [They're] storming forward with advances and I thought, 'I just don't know enough about this'. I didn't want to be hurried into a decision and I think at the time they were saying . . . it was going to be used to find out, for research on asthma and I felt terribly guilty saying 'no' because I had four healthy children and I appreciate how lucky I am, my husband's healthy and I'm healthy . . . but I still didn't feel as if I could say 'yes' because I just didn't.
>
> (M056)

She said she wanted to protect her baby but could not do so if she donated to NCCGP as she had no control over what was done to the samples. Lack of control was cited in several accounts as a reason for not donating, rather than not wanting to help. One said, 'I feel like I've got some paranoid conspiracy thing going on but there you go. It's with not knowing anything about it, I suppose. I find that really spooky' (M035).

Another said:

Before I had a child of my own, it was just a general concern about the database and what they might abuse in the future – that you might have very little control over that despite the best safeguards and the best intentions in the world. But when actually the child is there, it's their consent as well that you're giving . . . maybe it's being used for something you're not aware of and you don't know that you ought to withdraw your consent on such and such a day.

(M071)

There was no indication of any undue pressure from the research team to participate, except possibly in the one account of the woman who regretted donating (see M040 above) who was a somewhat 'reluctant participant'. This woman occupies an interesting position of ambivalence towards the database and raises more questions about why women do donate, posing this as the problematic question (rather than the question of why women refuse), and in so doing also sheds some interesting light on the tendency of the NCCGP's team to minimize the levels of involvement required by participation in the database:

It could be pressure from the midwife who may say something like, 'Oh, flaming donate! The placenta, it doesn't really matter, it just gets thrown in the bin anyway'. Do you know what I mean? Making the issue seem very small and insignificant. It would be the way that it's actually put over when you have an antenatal visit or whatever. Maybe people don't think about things, the possibility that it could lead to something they don't want, so maybe people are too trusting. I mean there is lots of reasons, isn't there? Maybe people feel guilty . . . There is lots of reasons why they would [donate].

(M040)

These accounts suggest that non-participants feel a generalized cultural pressure or imperative to donate and to help which is perhaps particularly acute during pregnancy when they are recipients of much medical help and support. It is often the case that those who are identified as deviating from the norm articulate most clearly what those norms are, in explaining their reasons for deviating and it might be that all the women felt this as a cultural pressure, even if they did not feel it as a direct pressure from the team. This suggests that participants and non-participants draw upon the same cultural framework in making their decisions about participation even if their actual levels or styles of participation differ.

Thus, we can suggest that as well as there being degrees of participation there are also styles of participation. For example, the 'active' participant, who is keen to make a contribution; and the 'cost/benefit' participant who balances the cost to themselves and their baby, which is seen as almost negligible against the benefit that their contribution might make to others. This in contrast is seen as being high, particularly in light of the potential eradication of disease. We also have identified the 'passive' participant who shrugs their shoulders and cannot really see any reason not to donate, and the 'reluctant' participant, of whom there was only one case. Most women appear to belong to the second category.

In some ways these data suggest that the NCCGP team have a fairly good picture of how the mothers regard the project. However, the combination of the two strands, often linked in the same sentence as we have seen, suggests that attributing full or partial participation to altruism is perhaps misplaced or at least overstated. Overall it appears that most mothers decided to help because it cost them very little to do so. Only one woman mentioned feeling that one ought to help whatever the cost:

> I hope that is the sort of attitude my children will have, you know if there is a way to help out without it causing any problems to them, then why not. You know, one step further than that, even if you're called on to help out somebody and it does cause you problems, you still go ahead and do it . . .
>
> (M034)

This perhaps is truly altruistic participation. It is important though to note that, as we have seen, non-participants display altruistic values too but consider the costs of donating to be just too high. In this way they are close in their attitudes to the costs/benefits participants mentioned above and therefore we can also see that there are not such strong distinctions between full or partial participants and non-participants as might at first be expected. This is an important point to make since it is often implicit in the claims about the altruistic motives of participants in genetic databases or in medical research in general that those who do not participate do not share the same altruistic attitudes. From the data presented here we would suggest that those who do participate are not necessarily as altruistic as is usually assumed and that those who do not participate are as equally altruistic as their participating counterparts.

The broader context of participation and non-participation

The material in all four sets of interviews (the NCCGP team, the community opposition, the participating mothers and the non-participating mothers) suggests that all the parties are constructing themselves as 'ethical beings' (Haimes and Wong Barr 2003). That is to say, they are all keen to demonstrate that they are acting in morally acceptable ways. The research team show that they are acting with integrity in not pressing women to donate to the project;

the opposition groups demonstrate that they can understand the imperative to help medical research, even though they oppose the way this has been funded; the mothers demonstrate that they are individuals who can appreciate the need to help, as a way of contributing to the welfare of others. Each version of 'being ethical' reflects the relevant context in which each interviewee is acting (Baruch 1981, Silverman 2001: 105–110). None of the interviewees referred to an overarching set of ethical principles to explain their own actions. Although they did to explain the actions of others, for example the way in which altruism is used to explain mothers' actions. This feature of the interviews is reminiscent of Foucault's interest in 'practices of the self' and the ways in which individuals construct themselves ethically 'without recourse to over-riding moral norms' (Osborne 1994: 487, Foucault 1997: 255–256, Haimes 2002) and Osborne's adaptation of Foucault's work in his concept of 'ethical stylizations'. This refers to the ways in which individuals within certain social contexts construct and sustain an acceptable sense of self, the acceptability itself being based on certain social and cultural frameworks for particular groups. Osborne argues that we now have a world of many ethical stylizations, but with few rules about ethical content (Osborne 1998: 221–231).

Tied to this is the absence of competing normative statements that we expected to find, particularly between the NCCGP team and the community opposition. The interviewees seem to suggest that it is morally inappropriate to say what others should do in particular circumstances. Another feature of the mothers' interviews was that none agreed with the suggestion that people ought to be made to donate to genetic databases, even though all might benefit, but rather they thought that individuals should be allowed to decide for themselves what the appropriate actions to take should be. This displays a broader cultural attitude that seems to suggest that everyone has to decide their own individual moral code rather than follow a set of prescribed behaviours. Giddens expresses this as one of the difficulties of what he labels the 'life politics' of late modernity, in which individuals no longer have the certainties of traditional society to guide their actions (1991: 214–224). For Bauman this is simply the reality of everyday life, though one which, he argues, most individuals manage without too much difficulty (1993: 32).

However, in the context of the NCCGP, this raises further questions. In identifying the nuanced understandings that shape the processes, levels and styles of participation, it is important not to forget two other groups that have a role in the NCCGP study, namely the children whose umbilical cord samples are seen as the central donation (in so far as provision of this constitutes, for the NCCGP, participation and non-provision constitutes non-participation) and the 'community' which features so prominently in the very name of the genetic database itself. So far, the children are silent and the community invisible, despite its apparent prominence. Both require some consideration if we are to understand fully what 'participation' and 'non-participation' in the NCCGP mean. Whilst there is insufficient space in this chapter to consider each in detail, each raises further questions about levels and styles of participation and non-participation that puts the data presented thus far in a broader social context.

The first point to raise is that, having heard the voices of some of those involved in the NCCGP, we are very aware that there are 'silent participants' whose voices have yet to be heard. There is a question of who has a voice in these debates about genetic databases and who remains or is forced to remain silent? In particular the voices of the children who have also donated to the NCCGP will not be heard for quite some time (see Williamson *et al.*, this volume, for a discussion of children's participation in this form of research). They are passive participants in the project in a particularly stark way. This is an issue that will need to be revisited as these children grow up into teenage-hood and adulthood, since their rights need to be considered. The NCCGP are clear that the children will be able to withdraw their samples once they reach the age of 16, but until then they are essentially silent donors whose materials will contribute to medical research but without their consent (see also Laurie 2000, 2001). Clearly this relates to other debates within medical ethics on the ability of children to consent to research, but its importance here needs to be remembered. To what extent do they have choices, now or in the future, about their levels of participation and to what extent will they later on reflect their mothers' styles of participation?

The very title of the NCCGP emphasizes both the location of the project (although in fact it is located in West Cumbria rather than North Cumbria) and characterizes that geographical location as a 'community'. This reveals another question for these discussions, which is how 'the community' is characterized. Why have these elements been included in the title rather than, for example, the purpose of the project or its desired outcomes? The analytical question to ask about this then is what does that use of the location, and its association with the notion of community, achieve? However deliberate or otherwise the choice of these terms has been, the effect of this use is to suggest a degree of participation and indeed ownership of the project by the community, which in turn suggests that they might be assumed to be the main beneficiaries of that project. However, community participation, even if deemed laudable, is both difficult to define and difficult to achieve. Its most common manifestation is through community consultation, but the ability to consult a community is an issue that remains a challenge for anyone involved in genetics research. The NCCGP undertook a series of public meetings to try to ensure that the community was informed about the project and there are varying accounts about the success of these meetings. Added to this is the need for a more critical approach to the term 'consultation', which implies a one-way relationship between two distinct parties. It is difficult for a community to enter into such a process since this is always likely to be a process of talking, in fact, with representatives of that community. How they are selected and how the consultation occurs is underpinned by political processes which in turn underpin the ways in which ethical issues are handled (Marinetto 2003). Therefore, even if the term consultation is replaced with a perhaps more evenly balanced and active term such as 'dialogue', the problem of just who has a voice in that dialogue remains.

Notions of 'community consent' are being raised as a way of trying to establish the acceptability, or otherwise, of projects such as the NCCGP. However, not only are there the questions already raised of who or what counts as the relevant community, there are also questions of how democratic this initially attractive notion might be. For example, in the NCCGP it could be argued that the donating groups, mothers and babies, are in fact socially vulnerable groups in any community and thus even if 'a community' gives its consent to their role as donors this might be open to abuse if those sectors do not have equal standing in that community. We know from much sociological work on this concept that communities are neither necessarily benign nor united, let alone protective of their most vulnerable members.

This however returns us to our starting point, to ask questions not just of the genetics research but also of this sort of sociological research that we have been conducting on projects such as the NCCGP. In seeking accounts from the women who have been approached by the NCCGP several things are happening. First, in asking the women to participate in interviews about their decision we are asking them for accounts of what they did and why. And in doing that, we are not just asking them for accounts, we are also asking them to be accountable for their actions (see also Hoeyer this volume). As we have seen, this process asks them to account for themselves as moral beings. Therefore in engaging with 'the public', as one strategy for making science accountable, are we in danger of putting the public under scrutiny and making them accountable too? And if so, is there a danger that they might be found wanting in some way; just as we have had the 'deficit model' in the public understanding of science, might we start to move towards a deficit model of moral behaviour? For example, might these data on the levels and styles of participation be used to try to develop 'better' ways of participating in genetic databases, such as UK Biobank? Might these variations be studied in order then to develop techniques for ensuring that most participants are of the 'fully participant, active' variety, such that other styles and levels are seen as morally inadequate? The notion of a citizen's duty to assist in medical research is gaining greater attention, but since, as we have seen here, participation is not necessarily accompanied by a greater understanding of what is being asked for, or why, there are dangers in pursuing such a style and level of participation as a single goal. These broader questions are rarely raised within ethical or policy related discussions around genetic databases (Jones and Salter 2003) and yet we would argue that they are just as important as many of the more commonly raised issues.

Conclusion

In conclusion then, 'participation' and 'non-participation' are not two clear categories; there are clear variations in both level and style. These variations are more marked than is usually supposed and reflect the social and moral contexts within which the request to donate was experienced. An important aspect of the social context is the situation in which the request to donate was made and how this affects the level and types of knowledge held about the donations given. Clearly this was an important aspect of the donors' perspective (did they even know they were donating?), but also, significantly, from the research team's perspective the question remains about how much it matters that the oft-quoted participation rate of 80–90 per cent was actually only a partial participation rate. That is, the lack of knowledge or potential lack of knowledge is not just a feature of lay people's understanding but also of the scientists' perspective. This is often either not noticed or ignored yet it is actually a key feature of much of the work around genetic databases, since they involve a great deal of ignorance and uncertainty about what data matter because, by their very nature, it is not clear what data and analysis will be needed by future studies making use of the database. We need to acknowledge this, rather than overplay levels of ignorance amongst lay groups and the public and underplay that amongst scientific researchers. An important aspect of the moral context is the degree of similarity between all groups as to how their levels and styles of participation both reflect and constitute their ethical reasoning, both about themselves and about their relationship to others. What is also clear from these interviews is that our understanding of interviewees' moral positions about participation and non-participation is necessarily filtered through our understanding of the social processes that shape the levels and styles of participation.

Acknowledgements

We are grateful to the Wellcome Trust, without whom this research would not have been possible. The authors would also like to acknowledge the additional support provided by Pat Spallone and Martin Sexton.

References

Baruch, G. (1981). 'Moral tales: parents' stories of encounters with the health profession', *Social Health and Illness* 3: 275–296.

Bauman, Z. (1993). *Postmodern Ethics*, Oxford: Blackwell.

Berger, A. (2001). 'UK genetics database plans revealed', *British Medical Journal* 322: 1018.

Beskow, L., Burke, W., Merz, J. *et al*. (2001). 'Informed consent for population-based research involving genetics', *Journal of the American Medical Association* 286: 2315–2321.

Chase, D., Tawn, E., Parker, L., Jonas, P. and Burn, J. (1998). 'The North Cumbria Community Genetics Project', *Journal of Medical Genetics* 35: 413–416.

Chase, D., Tawn, E., Parker, L., Jonas, P. and Burn, J. (2000). The North Cumbria Community Genetics Project 1996–2000. Unpublished interim report: Westlakes Research Institute and University of Newcastle.

Clarke, A. (1998). *The Genetic Testing of Children*, Oxford: BIOS.

Cragg Ross Dawson (2000). Public perceptions of the collection of human biological samples. Report prepared for the Wellcome Trust and Medical Research Council.

EPEG Project (2001). Ethical Protection in Epidemiological Genetic Research: Participants' Perspectives. Interim report. Centre for Ethics in Medicine, University of Bristol.

Foucault, M. (1997). 'On the genealogy of ethics: an overview of work in progress', in P. Rabinow (ed.) *Michel Foucault: Ethics, Subjectivity and Truth*, London: Allen Lane, pp. 255–256.

Garcia, J. (ed.) (1990). *The Politics of Maternity Care*, Oxford: Clarendon Press.

Giddens, A. (1991). *Modernity and Self-Identity*, Cambridge: Polity Press, pp. 14–224.

Gustafsson-Stolt, U., Liss, P., Svensson, T. and Ludvigsson, J. (2002). 'Attitudes to bioethical issues', *Social Science and Medicine* 54: 1333–1344.

Haimes, E. (2002). 'What can the social sciences contribute to the study of ethics?' *Bioethics* 16: 89–113.

Haimes, E. and Whong-Barr, M. (2003). 'Competing perspectives on reasons for participation and non-participation in the North Cumbria Community Genetics Project', in B.M. Knoppers (ed.) *Populations and Genetics: Legal, Socio-ethical Perspectives*, Leiden: Brill Academic Publishers, pp. 199–216.

Hansard (2002). Biobank. *Houses of Parliament* (2002): 365–372.

House of Lords Select Committee on Science and Technology (2000). Science and society, 3rd report, London: The Stationery Office.

House of Lords Select Committee on Science and Technology (2001). Human genetic databases, 4th report, London: The Stationery Office.

Human Genetics Commission (2000). 'Whose hands on your genes?' A discussion document on the storage, protection and use of personal genetic information. London: Human Genetics Commission.

Human Genetics Commission (2002). Inside information: Balancing interests in the use of personal genetic data. London: Human Genetics Commission.

Jacobus M. (1990). *Women and the Discourses of Science*, London: Routledge.

Jones, M. and Salter, B. (2003). 'The governance of human genetics: policy discourse and construction of public trust', *New Genetics and Society* 22: 21–41.

Kaye, J. and Martin, P. (2000). 'Safeguards for research using large scale DNA collections', *British Medical Journal* 321: 1146–1149.

King, D. (2000). A democratic model for research using gene banks. Submission to House of Lords Select Committee on Science and Technology. Written evidence on genetic databases.

Laurie, G. (2000). 'Genetics and patients' rights: where are the limits?' *Medical Law International* 5: 25–44.

Laurie, G. (2001). 'Challenging medical-legal norms: the role of autonomy, confidentiality and privacy in protecting individual and familial group rights in genetic information', *Journal of Legal Medicine* 22: 1–54.

Lowrance, W. (2001). 'The promise of human genetic databases', *British Medical Journal* 322: 1009–1010.

Marinetto, M. (2003). 'Who wants to be an active citizen? The politics and practice of community involvement', *Sociology* 37: 103–120.

Martin, P. (2000). The industrial development of human genetic databases. Submission to the House of Lords. Written evidence on genetic databases. House of Lords, 1999–2000.

Mason, J. and McCall Smith, A. (1999). *Law and Medical Ethics*, 5th edn, London: Butterworths.

Meade, T. and Hopkinson, I. (2001). 'Safeguards for research using large scale DNA collections', *British Medical Journal* 322: 551.

O'Neill, O. (2002). 'Some limits of informed consent', *Journal of Medical Ethics*, 28: 0–3.

Osborne, T. (1994). 'Sociology, liberalism and the historicity of conduct', *Economy and Society* 23: 484–501.

Osborne, T. (1998). 'Constructionism, authority and the ethical life', in I. Velody and R. Williams (eds) *The Politics of Constructionism*, London: Sage, pp. 221–234.

Rose, H. (2000). The commodification of bioinformation: the Icelandic health sector database. Wellcome Trust.

Silverman, D. (2001). *Interpreting Qualitative Data*, 2nd edn, London: Sage, pp. 105–110.

Spallone, P. and Wilkie, T. (2000). 'The research agenda in pharmacogenetics and biological sample collections', *New Genetics and Society* 19: 193–205.

Staley, K. (2001). Giving your genes to Biobank UK: questions to ask. Genewatch UK.

Voss, G. (2000). Report to the Human Genetics Commission on public attitudes to the use of human genetic information, London: Human Genetics Commission.

Wade, N. (2002). 'A genomic treasure hunt may be striking gold', *New York Times*, 18 June.

Weisbrot, D. (2003). 'The Australian joint inquiry into the protection of human genetic information', *New Genetics and Society* 22: 89–113.

Whong-Barr, M. (2002). 'Consent: a matter of form over substance? The case of British and US population-based genetic research'. Paper presented to 'Next Generation of Leaders in Science and Technology Policy' Research Symposium, Washington D.C., November 2002.

Chapter 5

Informed consent

The contradictory ethical safeguards in pharmacogenetics

Oonagh Corrigan

Introduction

Since the late 1990s, an increasing number of DNA samples are being collected from patients and healthy volunteers participating in clinical drug trials, to be used for genetics research. This type of research is being carried out globally, usually at the instigation of large multinational pharmaceutical companies, many of which are building extensive genetic databases. While there has been a great deal of attention to and debate surrounding the collection of DNA samples for use in public genetic databases, there has been virtually no discussion of the formation of such databases being compiled on behalf of or by the pharmaceutical industry (see Lewis this volume). This is somewhat surprising given that much of the debate surrounding public databases concerns their potential commercial exploitation (Marks and Steinberg 2002). The systematic collection of samples by industry is linked to what is known broadly as pharmacogenomic research and first began to appear in the form of 'add on' studies to the main drug trial protocol in the late 1990s. 'Pharmacogenomics' is the name given to a broad-based pharmaceutical industry-led initiative, based on developments brought about by the Human Genome Project which aims to capitalize on this knowledge base to discover new therapeutic targets and interventions and to elucidate the constellation of genes that determine the efficacy and toxicity of specific medications. 'Pharmacogenetics' is a more specific term used to define the narrower spectrum of inherited differences in drug metabolism and disposition linked to individual genetic variations. The pharmaceutical industry is currently focusing their research efforts on the latter (using DNA collected during clinical trials), while also storing samples longer term for as yet unspecified pharmacogenomics research. Many large pharmaceutical companies are now engaged in genomic-based research and making substantial financial investment in this area.[1] Industry-sponsored clinical drug trials take place on a global scale, with perhaps several thousand patients worldwide simultaneously taking part in any single clinical trial.[2] Drug development is an extremely time consuming and costly operation, taking 10–15 years and costing an estimated

US$300–600 million with a success rate of about 1 in 10, only a fraction of which will be 'blockbusters'. Development of new blockbuster drugs is becoming increasingly difficult (Horrobin 2000) and pharmacogenomics promises revolutionary forms of drug development with substantial financial gains for the industry:

> Industry analysts predict that, by improving medical outcomes by the use of pharmacogenomics-enhanced drugs and diagnostics, pharmaceutical companies could benefit to the order of US$200 million to US$500 million in extra revenue for each drug. . . . For these reasons, pharmaceutical companies have begun to integrate pharmacogenomics into drug development programs.
>
> (Bogdanovic and Langlands 1999: 182)

The collection of blood samples for pharmacogenomics-related studies first began to be added to clinical drug trials during the late 1980s. While it is difficult to get an accurate assessment of the scale of such research (see Lewis this volume) a company director of one of Europe's main laboratories conducting pharmacogenetic tests informed me that in the year 2000 his company had handled 12,000 samples, half of which were from UK drug companies and that there are at least two other such laboratories operating in Europe. Furthermore, he hinted at the global scale of these tests:

> [W]e [the Clinical Research Company that owns this laboratory] don't just do it for Europe, we do it on a global basis. So we've got a lab in the States, we've got a lab in Australia in Sydney, another lab in Cape Town South Africa, and a lab in Singapore.

Some pharmaceutical companies are taking quite a targeted approach and are engaged in collecting samples from patients in specific clinical trials. For example, one of the world's largest pharmaceutical companies is targeting selected conditions such as metabolic disorders and during an interview with one of the clinical genetic scientists from this company I was informed of genetic tests being carried out on a particular multinational trial for a drug to treat type II diabetes involving 11 trials in Europe and the US and 4000 patients. What distinguishes this type of genetic data collection from other forms of regional or national databases is its global dimension and its lack of public knowledge of or accountability for research carried out on commercial databases. The numbers of patients enrolled in such trials worldwide are increasing and a recent article published in the *New England Journal of Medicine* urges the collection of 'genomic DNA from all patients enrolled in clinical drug trials, along with appropriate consent to pharmacogenetic studies' (Evans and McLeod 2003: 547).

The collection of blood samples for this form of research has been facilitated by the pre-existing ethical regulatory mechanisms that govern the conduct of conventional clinical drug trials. A range of governance mechanisms are in place, in the form of national and international ethical codes and systems of 'independent' ethical review, and are based on the ethical requirement to obtain the informed consent of research subjects, and weigh the risks and benefits of participation in research. Informed consent in particular is an ideal that has gained increasing salience within Western healthcare policy, having become progressively something of an ethical panacea since it first emerged over fifty years ago in international guidelines governing biomedical research (Corrigan 2003). In pharmacogenomics-related clinical drug trials, consent is first sought from subjects to take part in the main clinical drug trial and, if they agree, they are subsequently asked to consent to the additional genetic aspect of the trial. In addition, subjects are informed that the sponsoring pharmaceutical company has sole property rights over the sample and the research results. This chapter, based on research supported by the UK's Wellcome Trust, examines the social and ethical implications of the development of pharmacogenetics in clinical trials and focuses on the issue of consent to these trials and the problems and contradictions surrounding this process.

The origins and compulsion of informed consent

Informed consent is based on the principle that competent individuals are entitled to choose freely whether to participate in research. Informed consent protects the individual's freedom of choice and respects the individual's autonomy.

(Council for International Organizations of Medical Sciences 1993)

During the past fifty years, the principle of informed consent, which has its roots in Western medicine and liberal theory (Beauchamp and Childress 1989, Burgess 2001) has become a cornerstone of contemporary biomedical research ethics, and been enshrined in a multitude of national and international ethics guidelines supported by mechanisms to ensure its adherence. Bioethicists writing on the historical emergence and development of clinical research ethics (Gray 1975, Faden and Beauchamp 1986, Beauchamp and Childress 1989, Annas and Grodin 1992, Katz 1992) point to a number of significant events occurring between the years preceding the Second World War and the end of the 1970s, which they claim have raised ethical concerns among those within the medical field and beyond. Furthermore, they claim that such concern has prompted the implementation of new policies, guidelines, and the general proliferation of a bioethics literature as now exists, to ensure ethical practice in clinical research involving human subjects. The field of research ethics in this context is constructed as progressive, concerned with checking the excesses of medical science and protecting the individual research subject from exploitation and harm.

The first critical event often cited is the emergence of evidence about horrific scientific and medical experiments conducted by Nazi physicians and scientists on prisoners during the Second World War. The *Nuremberg Code* (1947), constituted in direct response to the exposure of these details during the trials of the Nazi doctors, at the end of the war, was the first major international ethical statement to stipulate principles of biomedical research. It consists of ten principles, the first of which stipulates that 'the voluntary consent of the human subject is absolutely essential'; this principle has become the primary ethical consideration in all biomedical research (Annas and Grodin 1992). A year after the *Nuremberg Code*, a more general response to the inhumanities of Nazism was established in the *Universal Declaration of Human Rights*. The requirement of informed consent was declared a universal human right, grounded in the fundamental dignity and worth of every individual and supported by respect for the liberty and security of the person. In 1954, the World Medical Association (WMA) adopted a set of ethical principles that went beyond the *Nuremberg Code*, and further extended the principle of informed consent to include surrogate consent for incapacitated subjects. The WMA followed this in 1964 with the *Declaration of Helsinki*, a more comprehensive set of guidelines, which, while further emphasizing the principle of consent, also included a distinction between therapeutic and non-therapeutic research. Nevertheless, despite the production of these and other national professional guidelines, in practice, informed consent procedures were not initially generally implemented or adhered to consistently.

The problem of non-compliance was highlighted by two whistle-blowers, Henry Beecher in the US and Maurice Pappworth in the UK, who produced documented evidence of cases where patients had been subject to medical research without their knowledge or consent (Beecher 1966, Pappworth 1967). Beecher described the now renowned Tuskegee case, a study lasting over forty years (1932–1972) and involving nearly four hundred black men from Tuskegee, Alabama, suffering from syphilis. These men were told they were being treated for 'bad blood' and enrolled in the study to observe the manifestations of syphilis. However, the study team went to great lengths to ensure that these men were not informed of the true nature of their condition or given penicillin, which by 1947 had been shown to cure the disease. The publication of this and other cases revealed by Beecher and Pappworth prompted implementation of further protective mechanisms to ensure adherence to informed consent procedures.[3]

During the 1970s, research ethics committees in the UK and 'institutional review boards' (IRBs) in the US were established to oversee research programmes and enforce compliance with international and professional ethics guidelines. The principal mandate of these committees was and continues to be the review of proposals to carry out research on patients or healthy volunteer subjects within the medical environment. These bodies act as gate-keepers to safeguard the welfare of subjects in clinical trials, ensure that prior written informed consent is obtained from patients, and that risk to subjects involved in biomedical research is minimized. Research ethics guidelines have continued to be updated over the last 30 years, and new ones have emerged to meet the changing terrain of medical research. The extent to which research ethics has been internalized by the commercial side of science and medicine is evidenced in a pharmaceutical industry-led initiative which has produced the most recent set of international policy guidelines promoting ethical standards in the context of clinical drug research (ICH 1998).[4] These guidelines promote an international ethical and scientific quality standard for designing, conducting, recording and reporting trials that involve the participation of human subjects, and claim consistency with the principles that have their origin in the *Declaration of Helsinki*. Great emphasis is again given to the concept of written 'fully informed consent', as well as specific stipulations about the nature of information that is mandatory for the researcher to disclose to the subject.

Interestingly, while ethics guidelines draw a distinction between therapeutic and non-therapeutic research, no distinction is drawn between commercial and non-commercial research. Such guidelines have emerged in almost complete absence of any real debate about the particular ethical issues that arise from pharmaceutical or other commercially sponsored clinical trials. Despite a number of recent articles published in the medical and bioethics literature highlighting the potential conflicts of interests of pharmaceutical-sponsored research (Steflox *et al.* 1998, Glass and Lemmens 1999), with the exception of guidance recommending that healthy subjects in taking part and physicians conducting such research are not unduly financially rewarded, there is at present no formal guidance for research ethics committees regarding such research.

Calculations of risk and benefit

The significance awarded to the principle of informed consent in biomedical research cannot be overstated. However, as I have already mentioned, the governance mechanisms in biomedical research also draw on a risk–benefit calculation. Research ethics committees are required both to scrutinize informed consent procedures and to ensure there is a correct balance between the potential risks and benefits. The following extract from the newly updated *Declaration of Helsinki* illustrates the kinds of risk–benefit considerations that those involved in conducting clinical research are required to adhere to:

> Every medical research project involving human subjects should be preceded by careful assessment of predictable risks and burdens in comparison with foreseeable benefits to the subject or to others. . . . Physicians should abstain from engaging in research projects involving human subjects unless they are confident that the risks involved have been

adequately assessed and can be satisfactorily managed. . . . Medical research involving human subjects should only be conducted if the importance of the objective outweighs the inherent risks and burdens to the subject. . . . Medical research is only justified if there is a reasonable likelihood that the populations in which the research is carried out stand to benefit from the results of the research.

(World Medical Association 2000)

Furthermore, most guidelines also draw a distinction between therapeutic and non-therapeutic research, highlighting the necessity to ensure that in non-therapeutic research, risks to subjects are minimized. This is premised on the notion that an individual taking part in a therapeutic study at least has the chance of benefiting by receiving treatment, and thus it may be deemed reasonable for the individual to be subjected to a higher degree of risk than a subject taking part in a non-therapeutic study where there is no such potential benefit. For example, a subject's involvement in pharmacogenetics research is non-therapeutic and therefore, as I will subsequently discuss, has implications for the ways in which risk is assessed. Current European legislation requires research ethics committees to ensure that written information given to the prospective research subject includes explanations of twenty different aspects relating to the subject's involvement in the trial (ICH 1998). These include explanations of the 'purpose of the trial', the trial procedures to be followed, the 'reasonably foreseeable risks' or inconvenience to the subject, and responsibilities the subject undertakes as a result of involvement in the trial. Nevertheless, while physicians and research ethics committees are required to ensure that risks and benefits are carefully assessed, ultimately it is the prospective research subjects themselves who are obliged to assess the risks and benefits.

> When a patient gives consent to participate in a piece of research he should have been given enough information to make his own choice. The concept of risk/benefit analysis should be conveyed to patients as part of the procedure of seeking consent.
>
> (Royal College of Physicians 1990:11)

Although research ethics committees have the dual task of scrutinizing informed consent procedures and ensuring that there is a correct balance between the potential risks and benefits, in practice most research ethics committees in the UK and Institutional Review Boards (IRBs) in the US give more priority and attention to informed consent procedures rather than the analysis of risks and potential benefit.[5] In effect, research ethics committees manage risk–benefit considerations by facilitating the process of informed consent and ensuring that sufficient written information is given to the patient or healthy volunteer subject, and includes details of the anticipated risks and benefits so that the subject may assess the risk and choose whether or not to participate.

The establishment of international and national ethical codes of practice such as the major ones I have highlighted, and the policies and practices that have arisen to ensure their implementation, are most often understood as a progressive response to the growing awareness of the need for regulation to protect subjects in clinical research. The public revelation of the atrocities committed by the Nazis, the cases exposed by Beecher and Pappworth, and the growing attention placed on human rights issues during the 1960s have all been cited as major contributory factors in the emergence of regulatory practices and policies on clinical research. Couched within the discourse of human rights and liberal principles based on respect for autonomy, the concept of informed consent is presented in regulatory guidelines and has been adopted in health research policy as the optimal ethical solution to mitigate the dangers of exploitation and coercion of the research subject. Patient advocacy groups have also welcomed the growing recognition of the need for informed consent. For example, the UK charity patient group Consumers for Ethics in Research (CERES) actively promotes the right to informed consent and inclusion of research subjects as 'partners' or 'participants' in clinical research (CERES 1999).

We can see then that the various techniques and procedures encompassed within the bioethical framework governing research rely on the constitution of an autonomous free thinking, rational subject who ultimately bears the responsibility for assessing risks and benefits. The mechanisms designed to protect subjects from harm and exploitation do so by 'empowering' subjects and giving them the right to make informed decisions about research participation. However, the right to autonomy comes with the concomitant obligation to make a rational choice about whether to consent, having first considered the information and made an assessment of the potential risks and benefits. And there is a parallel obligation on the part of researchers to provide sufficient information for subjects to make an informed decision. I suggest that the informed consent process can be understood as a process that in effect constructs subjects as 'biological citizens' who have rights to be informed about biomedical research, and who simultaneously have obligations to make informed, reflective choices.

The notion of active citizenship has become increasingly prominent in political discussions and policy practices in Britain in the past 15 years (Marinetto 2003). This is seen as a significant development insofar as conventional practices of modern liberal democracies have been based on a representative mode of government in which the wider citizenry has a more passive role. However, we need to acknowledge that such participatory forms of active citizenship place an onus upon subjects to engage with the informed consent process. Although citizens can opt-out of this obligation – either by refusing to engage in this process and decline trial participation, or by accepting study participation based on 'blind trust' or in deference to medical authority – in the context of participatory citizenship such an action is seen as morally 'invalid'. Biological, scientific and technological citizenship requires that 'valid public acceptance must be deep and informed, subjective, voluntary, rigorous, and rich. Invalid acceptance involves thoughtless deference and blind trust' (Frankenfeld 1992: 460). Underpinning this model of active citizenship is a notion of an autonomous, rational, free thinking moral being.

Governed through freedom

That 'medical progress is based on research which ultimately must rest in part on experimentation involving human subjects' (World Medical Association 2000) is an a priori and, as such, medical research involving human subjects continues to proliferate. Furthermore, the current ethical system premised on informed consent is one that must be understood as most readily fulfilling the prior requirement of neo-liberal society to conduct research for the sake of 'medical progress', while at the same time appealing to an individualistic notion of 'free choice' and the protection of autonomy. The concept of 'freedom' here is understood in conventional liberal political and moral philosophical terms to be a terrain that exists outside the field of power. 'Free will' as understood by Immanuel Kant is the domain of every rational, moral autonomous agent:

> If a rational subject supposed his judgements to be determined, not by rational principles, but by external impulsion, he could not regard these judgements as his own. This must equally be true of practical reason: a rational agent must regard himself as capable of acting on his own rational principles and only so he can regard his will as his own. That is to say, from a practical point of view every rational agent must presuppose his will to be free. Freedom is a necessary presupposition of all action as well as of thinking.
>
> (Kant 1995 [1948]: 40)

Libertarian philosophies too, such as those of John Stuart Mill, are concerned with the individuality of action and thought, and claim that people should be able to make their own choices and decisions, free from governmental intervention and control. However, I would argue that ideas such as 'freedom' and autonomy should not be understood as politically innocent premises.

Michael Foucault's genealogical approach reveals that power and knowledge are central components in the historical transformation of various 'regimes of truth'. His approach to the study of power rejects the traditional concept as one of an external dominating force possessed by one group over another. He offers instead a radically new concept of power, linking it inexorably to knowledge. In *The Birth of the Clinic*, Foucault (Foucault 1991 [1963]) charts the emergence at the end of the eighteenth century of what he calls the political anatomy of the body. Medicine, he argues, becomes an increasingly important vehicle for the exercise of surveillance and control, concerned with both 'anatomo-politics of the human body' and 'the bio-politics of the population'.[6] By this, Foucault means that the technologies of this disciplinary apparatus serve to fabricate discrete individuals and, at the same time, extend the constantly normalizing medical gaze over the whole population. Furthermore, Foucault's historical analysis highlights the ways in which various rationalities of modern government are not mere mechanisms of social control and subordination of the human will but rather operate through the promotion of certain kinds of subjectivities. Bodies become the objects through which these disciplinary mechanisms are exercised, not through overt violence and coercion, but through a micro-politics of discipline (Foucault 1991). Biomedical research involving human subjects is now subjected to regulatory mechanisms to ensure research is no longer based on direct coercion, but through an individual's freely given informed consent. Nikolas Rose (1996) and others who have followed Foucault's line of analysis demonstrate the extent to which governmentality forges the modern embodied individual subject.[7] Rose highlights the way that, in advanced liberal society, the subject is situated in relation to a host of technologies and strategies aimed at governing through the regulated and accountable choices of autonomous agents:

> Advanced liberal rule . . . does not seek to govern through 'society', but through the regulated choices of individual citizens, now constructed as subjects of choices and aspirations to self-actualization and self-fulfilment. Individuals are to be governed through their freedom.
>
> (Rose 1996: 41)

I suggest that the individual human subject of biomedical research has been variously constructed. First, in the period prior to the adoption and implementation of ethical codes of practice, subjects were frequently constructed as passive, irrelevant or even as expendable objects of research who could be coerced or manipulated to take part. Second, the implementation of various protectionist measures and risk–benefit calculations constructs vulnerable subjects, subjects who need protecting from exploitation and harm. Finally, the increasing significance awarded to informed consent constructs subjects as empowered citizens who, given sufficient information, are able to make free, informed, rational and thus moral choices with respect to their participation. I suggest that such constructs obscure the extent to which subjects are treated and experience trial participation as all three. Furthermore, as I will discuss later in this chapter, none of these constructs encompasses the ways in which research subjects provide valuable labour and bodily material for pharmaceutical research, making them co-producers of drug products.

Clinical drug trials and sample collections: a multi-layered consent practice

As I have already indicated, currently blood samples for pharmacogenomics research purposes are being collected during otherwise conventional clinical drug research. Pharmaceutical companies' objectives towards the development of pharmacogenetics-based drug production are currently being pursued through studies of genetic variability in drug response. Pharmacogenetic tests are carried out to find correlations between an individual's drug-metabolizing enzymes and their response to the drug being taken. Pharmaceutical companies are also engaged with a wider range of research using collected DNA samples for the production of potential therapies based on an understanding of the genetics involved in individual susceptibility to disease.

New drugs developed by pharmaceutical companies are required to go through lengthy testing procedures before being granted a licence and made available for the general patient population. Following a period of lab testing including standard animal and *in vitro* tests, the new drug is tested in human subjects during several phases of clinical trials. At this stage, physicians are recruited by the sponsoring pharmaceutical company to act as 'trial investigators' and oversee the study and the administration of the drug according to the predetermined trial protocols. During phase I trials, the drug is tested on human subjects for the first time, and most of theses studies are conducted on healthy volunteer subjects in specially designated clinical trial suites (much like a private hospital ward).[8] Phase I studies are conducted either directly by the sponsoring pharmaceutical company in corporate premises, or the trials are subcontracted to specially designated clinical research organizations (CROs). Healthy volunteer subjects are financially rewarded for allowing their bodies to be used as experimental sites and most individuals taking part in such research do so primarily for economic gain (Corrigan 2000). Further phases of clinical drug trials (phases II to IV) involve greater numbers of subjects and are normally conducted on patients who suffer from the medical condition for which the test drug is an intended treatment. These studies are conducted in regular clinical settings such as hospital outpatient clinics, community clinics or GP surgeries and hospital wards. During these latter phases, patients are generally asked to participate in research by physicians during the course of routine clinical encounters.

Generally, drug trial subjects are asked to consent to three separate aspects of research. They are asked to consent to the main clinical drug trial, and then also to 'add-on' pharmacogenetic research in which they consent to an 'identified' genetic test for research related to drug effect, and a 'non-identified' test for unspecified future research. These three aspects are progressive insofar as giving consent to the second and third aspects is dependent on giving prior consent to the first and second. Patients being asked to take part in clinical drug trials are often given no prior notice about potential research but rather the possibility of participating in research is introduced during clinical consultation. This initial aspect of informed consent involves considerations relevant to participation in the drug trial itself. Subjects are given written and verbal information relating to the known risks of the drugs as well as details about procedures, such as the length of the study, the number of hospital visits required, and blood tests or X-rays associated with the study. In consenting to this first stage, patients agree to take part in a therapeutic drug trial and it is expected, as part of the consent process, that they will consider issues relating to the potential benefits and risks of the trial, including harms such as adverse drug reactions. Research examining the experiences of patients who have given their consent to take part in such trials demonstrates that despite the ethical rhetoric of informed consent based on adequate understanding of the information given to prospective subjects, in practice the reality is often very different. Despite the fact that patients are given information under headings such as 'possible risks' (usually relating to drug-induced side-effects), patients are often unable subsequently to recall the mention of any side-effects (Hassar and Weintraub 1976, Bergler *et al.* 1980, Cassileth *et al.* 1980, Estey *et al.* 1994).

Clinical drug trials are generally randomized so that neither the patient nor the medical team know whether a particular trial subject is taking the study drug, an alternative drug, or in some cases a placebo (a dummy pill). Studies show that trial subjects have poor understanding of the process of randomization in clinical drug trials (Cassileth *et al.* 1980, Jan and DeMets 1981, Snowdon *et al.* 1997), and as a consequence are sometimes under the misapprehension that they will be receiving an active treatment (Corrigan 2003). Furthermore, given the clinical context of these studies, from the perspective of the patient the boundaries between research and treatment are often quite fuzzy. In such circumstances, a request to consent is often interpreted as *guidance* to consent, insofar as patients have pre-existing expectations and norms regarding the role of the physician as a professional offering advice to patients about their best interests. Research in this area demonstrates that this so-called 'therapeutic misconception' is common (Bamberg and Budwig 1992, Dresser 2001). There is also evidence that some patients who consent to take part in clinical drug trials experience such decisions as 'burdensome' (Taylor 1988, Corrigan 2003); my own research indicates this is more likely to be the case for patients who have an acute condition or who are in pain or suffering great anxiety. Nevertheless, while research ethics guidelines recognize that for some patients giving 'adequate' consent might be difficult and such subjects are to be considered as 'vulnerable', these guidelines apply mainly to 'incompetent' subjects such as those who have some form of cognitive impairment (Council for International Organizations of Medical Sciences 1993, World Medical Association 2000). Such guidelines do not therefore address the varying needs of sick but otherwise competent patients. Although there is a growing awareness of problems relating to the practice of informed consent in clinical trials, solutions to such problems focus on improving written information given to patients, making sure that such information is comprehensive, detailing trial procedures and risks likely to be encountered by subjects (ICH 1998). In relation to consent to DNA tissue sample collections, here too problems and their solutions frequently centre on adequacy and comprehensiveness of information with solutions being proffered in terms of suggested comprehensively designed 'model' consent forms (Knoppers 1998, Merz and Sankar 1998). There is scant regard in both conventional bioethics guidelines and more socially nuanced policy perspectives of the need to appreciate more fully the social context in which consent is acquired. In the case of pharmacogenetics add-on studies to clinical drug trials, not only are patients being asked to consider complex issues related to the treatment of their condition and the potential risks and benefits of participating in the trial process, but they are further required to consider issues relating to the pharmacogenetics aspect of the trial.

In consenting to the second part of the study patients give the sponsoring pharmaceutical company permission to carry out genetic research on their blood sample, including linking it to personal medical information, such as details of their medical condition and family history. The sample at this stage is 'identified', meaning that the patient's name, medical history and DNA sample data all remain linked. According to an information leaflet produced by a pharmaceutical company to inform patients about such research: 'we will use the Identified Sample to look at genes that might be involved in the condition you have, and how those genes might affect the study medication you are receiving' (patient information leaflet 1998). Subjects are informed that samples will remain 'identified' for about six months after completion of the main drug trial study, and that such trials may take several years to complete. Indeed, patients may even be informed that their identified sample could be kept for up to a maximum of ten years.

The third part of the consent process involves a request to store the sample after completion of the trial for an unlimited period in order to carry out future, as yet unspecified, research. Subjects are informed that at this stage the sample will be 'non-identified'. By non-identified the pharmaceutical companies mean that the DNA sample, data derived from it and medical data concerning the subject will be stored but that it will not be possible to link this information to the name of the subject and as such anonymity will be secured. If subjects agree to consent to the third stage then identification markers linking the patient to the sample will be destroyed and the sample will be stored anonymously:

> [The pharmaceutical company], or people working with [the company] will store your blood sample (or genetic sample prepared from your blood). They will also store information about your medical history. After [the company] takes your identification off, they will store the sample,

all medical information, and any genetics results for an unlimited amount of time.

(patient consent form 1998)

The information given to patients and healthy volunteers is expected to be sufficient for making informed choices. However, unlike conventional clinical drug trials where information regarding potential risk relates mostly to the risk of bodily harm, apart from the slight possibility of bruising when a small blood sample is extracted from the subject, no other direct physical risks are involved in the pharmacogenetics aspect of the trial. Sponsoring pharmaceutical companies indicate that the risk of harm from participation in the genetic study is 'small' (patient information leaflet 1998). Risks are identified rather as relating to potential problems concerning confidentiality and anonymity. A patient information leaflet given to subjects gives assurances about sufficient measures in place to ensure that confidentiality and anonymity of this data are maintained. However, subjects are also informed that the pharmaceutical company 'cannot be certain that your genetic test results could never be linked to you' (patient information leaflet 1998). Although the risk of such harm is described as 'small', genetic information arising from such studies is potentially dangerous insofar as it may lead to discrimination in the workplace or difficulty in obtaining insurance if individuals are thought to have greater than average risk of ill-health. Indeed, an information video produced by the pharmaceutical company GlaxoSmithKline (GSK) aimed at informing clinical investigators about pharmacogenetic trials, emphasizes the need for doctors to ensure that the patient's privacy is protected. GSK representatives state that access to the data is to be restricted and such data must not be given to patients or insurers.

Insofar as consideration of potential benefits is concerned, unlike the main drug trial where patients may directly benefit as part of their involvement in the study, there is no likely direct benefit to the patient in taking part in the collection of samples for pharmacogenetics purposes. Whether or not patients in a clinical drug trial achieve the 'ideal' of autonomous decision-making, or they find the experience of consent empowering, there generally remains at least a potential therapeutic benefit to the patient in trial participation. Indeed, the hope of therapeutic effect is a reason often cited by patients for consenting to drug trials (Corrigan 2003). When clinical drug trials are non-therapeutic, as in the case of phase I trials conducted on healthy volunteers, subjects are financially rewarded for their participation. Other forms of non-therapeutic trials sometimes take place in the clinical setting, as for example in epidemiology or observational studies, but to my knowledge, these are not sponsored directly by pharmaceutical companies or other commercial organizations. Patients participating in pharmacogenetics research are not informed of the results of their genetic test even when such information may reveal that the patient is potentially a poor metabolizer for the study drug (or indeed for other drugs that rely on the same metabolizing enzyme) and thus are potentially at greater risk of experiencing adverse drug reactions. Instead, patients are informed that they are unlikely to benefit directly and an appeal is made to altruistic reasons for donation:

> [The pharmaceutical company] expects no immediate benefit to you although your participation in this research may eventually help people with migraine. . . . We may also learn which patients may suffer side-effects from certain medicines.
>
> (patient information leaflet 1998)

Risks to be considered for this aspect of the trial are deemed to be smaller insofar as at this stage it would not be possible for those involved in the trial to link the patient formally to the sample and the data. However, there remains a small risk that the patient could still be identified from the data relating their medical information with sample information, both of which remain linked. Furthermore, patients at this stage are consenting to as yet unspecified commercial research and have no future control over the kinds of research to which their samples may be used.

Should individuals not wish to consent to this third part of the study, they are informed that their sample will be removed and destroyed. However, as Graham Lewis (this volume) indicates, given the complex arrangements concerning storage of these samples by third party companies, many of whom are currently undergoing mergers, this endeavour may prove difficult and without effective oversight it may be hard to ascertain whether these promises are being adhered to.

Conclusion

In this chapter I have demonstrated that informed consent procedures have been introduced as a mechanism to protect the research subject's right to autonomy and appear to fit well with other strategies that encourage active forms of citizenship. Nevertheless, representing consenting patients as 'active participants' fails to acknowledge the extent to which they remain objects in the research process and are a potential vulnerable population. In the case of clinical drug trials where patients are not only being asked to consent to the main trial but are additionally being asked to consent to further pharmacogenetics-related studies, I suggest that the limits of consent are being overreached. Given evidence of the inability of patients who have decided to take part in clinical trials to comprehend information fully on trial procedures, along with their inability to recall information about potential risks, it is very unlikely that patients entering into pharmacogenetics-related trials will conform to the informed consent requirements of having given due careful consideration of all potential risks and benefits. As I have already indicated, consent is obtained in the clinical context, usually during consultations with a physician in the hospital or at an outpatient clinic. I suggest that asking patients to consent to further pharmacogenetics studies in this context is a form of exploitation, because they frequently already feel overburdened with information and anxiety, and in a weakened position to make independent decisions. Although in conventional clinical drug trials patients are subjected to additional risks over and above conventional therapy, insofar as there is only partial information on the efficacy and safety of the drug being tested in general, patients have at least the possibility of benefiting either from the comparative drug being tested or from the trial drug. However, as I have argued, there is no direct benefit to the patient in the pharmacogenetics study and thus compromises in the consent process cannot be offset against potential therapeutic benefit. This issue is of sufficient concern that in France, for example, non-therapeutic research is reviewed by different ethics review bodies from those reviewing therapeutic research, with the result that the conduct of pharmacogenetics add-on trials has been prevented.

More importantly, pharmaceutical companies, who have huge commercial incentives for developing genetic-based drugs, are sponsoring pharmaco-genetics trials. While physicians and medical professionals are involved in conducting the actual trials, pharmaceutical companies pay physicians for this service. Following the John Moore case (1998–1990), in which a cell line was patented and sold to the drug company Sandoz for $15 million, issues of property rights are increasingly being raised in relation to tissue samples (Boyle 1992, Landecker 1999). As such, blood samples that are donated for genetic testing purposes during the pharmacogenetic part of a clinical trial may potentially be extremely valuable commodities in genetic-based drug development. That said, human subjects have been experimental vessels for the production of drugs and subsequent commercial profit for well over half a century. In pharmacogenetic clinical trials, it is not simply the issue of DNA tissue that is at stake, but also human bodies and their labour, insofar as taking part in the trial may mean that the patient is required to attend the hospital clinic for tests related to the trial at regular intervals. Not only does the collection of DNA samples provide the 'raw material for industry' (see Lewis this volume) but trial subjects are also worked upon and transformed into data that are essential drug product components.

Such a conclusion raises profound questions about the meaning of consent for these trials. Should patients be financially rewarded for their involvement, as is the case for healthy subjects in phase I trials, as well as the physicians who recruit, conduct and oversee the clinical trials? Or should the fact that patients in the main trial are likely to receive benefit in the form of therapy be sufficient reward for taking part in all or some of the three aspects? And to what extent should altruistic reasons on the part of patients be taken into consideration? While pharmaceutical companies are foremost profit-making organizations and economic generators, they are also the vehicle by which successive governments have chosen to develop and test new drugs. We are thus left with the challenge of determining how to regulate clinical drug trials and pharmacogenetics research in a way that better protects patients and research subjects, but does not overly restrict potential medical breakthroughs. Of one thing we can be certain: informed consent is not a sufficiently robust concept (even were its implementation to be improved) to protect research subjects adequately – better protection is required if the risks that patients take as subjects in clinical trials are to be justified.

Acknowledgements

I would like to thank Jose Lopez, Martin Richards, Bryn Williams-Jones and Richard Tutton for their comments on earlier drafts of this chapter.

Notes

1. In 1998 the estimated pharmaceutical industry investment in genomics approached $2bn (Bogdanovic and Langlands 1999: 141).
2. For a more detailed description and information about the processes of each trial phase see Corrigan (2002).
3. Beecher (1966) compiled a list of more than twenty examples of unethical experiments, the results of which had been published in prestigious medical journals during a single year. Both Pappworth in the UK and Beecher in the US suggested that unethical research was widespread.
4. International Conference on Harmonisation (ICH 1998) is a pharmaceutical industry-led initiative aimed at standardizing good clinical practice (GCP) to provide a unified standard for the EU, Japan and the US.
5. A survey of 58 members belonging to six local research ethics committees in the UK area reveals that members rated their duty 'to ensure prospective subjects understand the implication of taking part in the study as the most important aspect of their work' (Kent 1997). This was given priority over and above the duty to protect subjects from harm. In the US IRBs have also been shown to prioritize informed consent over risk–benefit analysis (Weijer 2000).
6. These are concepts expanded more fully by Foucault (1979).
7. Governmentality studies focus on the technical character of liberal and neo-liberal government. This approach analyses the multi-form tactics of government, where the term 'government' is not to be understood simply in terms of the exercise of state power, but as a complex array of strategies of rule where techniques of power and domination interact with techniques of the self. For a comprehensive range of discussions on the concept of 'governmentality' by its various exponents see especially Barry et al. (1996).
8. Phase I trials are also conducted on patients with life-threatening conditions such as advanced or aggressive cancer.

References

Annas, G. and Grodin, M. (eds) (1992). *The Nazi Doctors and the Nuremberg Code*, New York: Oxford University Press.

Bamberg, M. and Budwig, N. (1992). 'Therapeutic misconceptions: when the voices of caring and research are misconstrued as the voice of curing,' *Ethics and Behaviour* 2: 165–184.

Barry, A., Osborne, T., and Rose, N. (1996). *Foucault and Political Reason*, London: The University of Chicago Press and UCL Press Limited.

Beauchamp, T.L. and Childress, J.F. (1989). *Principles of Biomedical Ethics*, Belmont: Wadsworth Publishing Company.

Beecher, H.-K. (1966). 'Ethics and clinical research,' *New England Journal of Medicine* 274: 1354–1360.

Bergler, J., Pennington, A., Metcalf, M., and Freis, E. (1980). 'Informed consent: how much does the patient understand?' *Clinical Pharmacology and Therapeutics* 27: 435–440.

Bogdanovic, S. and Langlands, B. (1999). *Pharmacogenomics Players*, London: Financial Times.

Boyle, J. (1992). 'A theory of information, copyright, spleens, blackmail and insider trading,' *California Law Review* 80: 1415–1540.

Burgess, M.M. (2001). 'Beyond consent: ethical and social issues in genetic testing,' *Nature Reviews: Genetics* 2: 9–14.

Cassileth, B., Zupkiss, R., Sutton-Smith, K., and March, V. (1980). 'Informed consent – why are its goals imperfectly realized?' *New England Journal of Medicine* 302: 896–900.

CERES (1999). *CERES News*. CERES (24).

Corrigan, O.P. (2000). Trial and error: a sociology of bioethics and clinical drug trials, unpublished PhD thesis, Department of Sociology, University of Essex.

Corrigan, O.P. (2002) 'A risky business: the detection of adverse drug reactions in clinical trials and post-marketing exercises', *Social Science and Medicine* 55 3: 497–507.

Corrigan, O.P. (2003). 'Empty ethics: The problem with informed consent,' *Sociology of Health and Illness* 25: 768–792.

Council for International Organizations of Medical Sciences (1993). International Ethical Guidelines for Biomedical Research Involving Human Subjects, Geneva: CIOMS.

Dresser, R. (2001). *When Science Offers Salvation: Patient Advocacy and Research Ethics*, Oxford: Oxford University Press.

Estey, A., Wilkin, G., and Dosseter, J. (1994). 'Are research subjects able to retain the information they are given during the consent process?' *Health Law Review* 3: 37–41.

Evans, W.E. and McLeod, H.L. (2003). 'Pharmacogenomics – drug disposition, drug targets, and side effects,' *New England Journal of Medicine* 348: 538–549.

Faden, R. and Beauchamp, T. (1986). *A History and Theory of Informed Consent*, New York: Oxford University Press.

Foucault, M. (1979). *The History of Sexuality*, London: Penguin.

Foucault, M. (1991). *Discipline and Punish*, London: Penguin.

Foucault, M. (1991 [1963]). *The Birth of the Clinic*, London: Routledge.

Frankenfeld, P.J. (1992). 'Technological citizenship: a normative framework for risk studies,' *Science Technology and Human Values* 17: 459.

Glass, K.C. and Lemmens, T. (1999). 'Conflicts of interest and commercialization of biomedical research', in T. Caulfield and B. Williams-Jones (eds), *The Commercialization of Genetic Research: Ethical, Legal and Policy Issues*, New York: Kluwer Academic/Plenum Press.

Gray, B.H. (1975). *Human Subjects in Medical Experimentation*, New York: John Wiley & Sons.

Hassar, M. and Weintraub, M. (1976). 'Uniformed consent and the wealthy volunteer: an analysis of patient volunteers in a clinical trial of a new anti-inflammatory drug,' *Clinical Pharmacology and Therapeutics* 29: 379–386.

Horrobin, D.F. (2000). 'Innovation in the pharmaceutical industry,' *Journal of the Royal Society of Medicine* 93: 341–345.

ICH (1998). International Conference for Harmonisation, Good Clinical Practice, Guidance for trials of medicinal products in the European Community, in C. Foster (ed.), *Manual For Research Ethics Committees*, London: Kings College, Centre of Medical Ethics and Law.

Jan, H. and DeMets, D. (1981). 'How informed is informed consent?' *Controlled Clinical Trials* 2: 287–303.

Kant, I. (1995 [1948]). *Groundwork of the Metaphysic of Morals*, London: Routledge.

Katz, J. (1992). 'The consent principle of the Nuremberg Code: its significance then and now,' in G. Annas and M. Grodin (eds), *The Nazi Doctors and the Nuremberg Code*, New York: Oxford University Press.

Kent, G. (1997). 'The views of members of Local Research Ethics Committees, researchers and members of the public towards the roles and functions of LRECs,' *Journal of Medical Ethics* 23: 186–190.

Knoppers, B.M. (1998). 'Human genetic material: commodity or gift?' in R.F. Weir (ed.), *Stored Tissue Samples: Ethical, Legal, and Public Policy Implications*, Iowa City: University of Iowa Press, pp. 226–235.

Landecker, H. (1999). 'Between beneficence and chattel: the human biological in law and science,' *Science in Context* 12: 203–225.

Marinetto, M. (2003). 'Who wants to be an active Citizen? The politics and practice of community involvement,' *Sociology* 37: 103–120.

Marks, A.D. and Steinberg, K.K. (2002). 'The ethics of access to online genetic databases: Private or public?' *American Journal of Pharmacogenomics* 2: 207–212.

Merz, J. and Sankar, P. (1998). 'DNA banking: an empirical study of a proposed consent form,' in R.F. Weir (ed.), *Stored Tissue Samples: Ethical, Legal and Public Policy Implications*, Iowa City: University of Iowa Press, pp. 198–225.

Pappworth, M. (1967). *Human Guinea Pigs*, Harmondsworth, UK: Pelican.

Rose, N. (1996). 'Governing "advanced" liberal democracies,' in A. Barry, T. Osborne and N. Rose (eds), *Foucault and Political Reason*, London: The University of Chicago Press and UCL Press Limited.

Royal College of Physicians (1990). *Research Involving Patients*, London: The Royal College of Physicians of London.

Snowdon, C., Garcia, J. and Elbourne, D. (1997). 'Making sense of randomization; responses of parents of critically ill babies to random allocation of treatment in a clinical trial,' *Social Science and Medicine* 45: 1337–1355.

Steflox, H.T., Chua, G., O'Rourke, K. *et al.* (1998). 'Conflict of interest in the debate over calcium channel antagonists,' *New England Journal of Medicine* 338: 101–106.

Taylor, K.M. (1988). 'Telling bad news: physicians and the disclosure of undesirable information,' *Sociology of Health and Illness* 10: 109–132.

Weijer, C. (2000). 'The ethical analysis of risk,' *Journal of Law, Medicine and Ethics* 28: 344–361.

World Medical Association (2000). Declaration of Helsinki: Ethical Principles for Medical Research Involving Human Subjects.

Chapter 6

Ambiguous gifts

Public anxiety, informed consent and biobanks

Klaus Hoeyer

Introduction

In 1999, a start-up biotech company called UmanGenomics acquired all commercial rights to Medical Biobank, a population-based research biobank in northern Sweden that contains blood samples collected since 1985 from a majority of the adult population in Västerbotten County.[1] When this arrangement was publicly announced, UmanGenomics made great play of its ethics policy, which was acclaimed in prestigious journals such as *Nature* (Abbott 1999) and *Science* (Nilsson and Rose 1999). At the time, this ethics policy contained three elements: informed consent procedures, an ethical review board and public control through majority ownership in the company by the county authorities and the local university.[2]

The ethics policy adopted by UmanGenomics reflects a wider trend by which the act of signing an informed consent form is the principal step in granting researchers access to blood derived from human beings (Beskow *et al.* 2001). Informed consent in relation to tissue donation is not yet an established routine. It can be seen as a relatively recent invention and, as such, confronts donors with partly new choices. These choices, I suggest, contribute to transformed perceptions of both the research that is conducted and the object that is donated. Given the emphasis in debates about informed consent on the informational content of consent forms both in the context of UmanGenomics and more broadly (Merz *et al.* 2003), one might expect donors' choices to be influenced by the information given in these forms. This appears not to be the case: few people remember or even read the consent form (Hoeyer 2003b). Many donors – and professionals working with the collection of blood – nevertheless hold strong views about genetic research and express anxieties concerning research they consider hazardous or wrong. That people have such opinions but apparently do not use the information offered to them about the research in which they are involved constitutes an empirical problem, a paradox so to speak, which I discuss in this chapter. This paradox is a starting point for exploring notions of anxiety and control in genetic research and the role that informed consent procedures play in relation to how anxiety and control is conceived and experienced by donors to Medical Biobank in Västerbotten.

The blood samples stored at the biobank, and used by UmanGenomics for its research, are procured at public healthcare centres. Everybody in Västerbotten County is invited for a medical examination at the ages of 40, 50 and 60 years. These examinations were initiated in Norsjö Municipality in 1985 in response to high mortality rates that were linked to a prevalence of cardiovascular diseases. It was known that some families were affected more than others, but the focus then was on factors that could be targeted by preventative interventions such as diet and lifestyle (Hallgren 1994, 1995). Several tools for public engagement in health issues were developed, including a labelling system of healthy foods that was subsequently adopted nationwide (Västerbottensprojektet 1991). After five years it was decided to offer the medical examinations across the whole county.

An examination takes a couple of hours and begins with some blood tests, during which the patients are asked whether they would like to donate 20 millilitres of blood for future research purposes. Until recently, an absolute majority have agreed to do so and willingly signed an informed consent form. A part of my research has involved observations of these examinations and interviews with 38 patients in a break, two-thirds of the way through their examinations. During the examinations I noticed how seldom people actually scrutinized the information before agreeing to donate this sample of blood for research. The donation takes place with relatively few words exchanged on the subject of the research in question (Hoeyer 2003b, Busby this volume). However, during the interviews most informants adopted a much more inquiring position, asking me questions, and stressing the importance of being properly informed and of being given the opportunity to refuse to participate in research. Some also conveyed their concern about rapid developments in the biosciences, particularly genetics.

In an attempt to understand this difference I argue that the donors' understanding of the substance they donate is ambiguous. The blood is *both* a few drops of blood of no consequence *and* important as 'part of' the donors. The informed consent form and my interviews are instances promoting the latter understanding, whereas the safety of being attended by a nurse promotes the former understanding. The implementation of informed consent procedures impinges on notions of self and personhood in ways that produce particular understandings of the donated blood and the individual's role in decision-making regarding its use. This is a complex matter that I address both with reference to the cultural specificities of Sweden and Västerbotten and the way that certain perceptions of personhood emerge through the informed consent procedures of this biobank and feature in informants' accounts of their donated blood or the genetic material derived from it. I further suggest that in the context of biobanks these procedures perform an ambiguous role of both limiting and producing anxiety.

First, I describe the medical examinations, the interviews I had with people attending the examinations, and the peculiar differences in tone between the two. I then turn to the question of public anxiety about genetic research, by considering the fears expressed about genetic research by biobank donors. I discuss notions of responsibility and causation: if there is fear and danger – who is responsible and how is control ensured? I suggest that a cultural understanding of the individual as a responsible actor, and control as being practically synonymous with public oversight and knowledge are both important issues in this Swedish case. This leads to a discussion of the role of informed consent procedures in relation to notions of anxiety and control. Rather than present one specific interpretation, this chapter provides several competing readings of the process of consent, thereby rendering a more complex understanding of informed consent procedures as dubious sites for the experience and production of both anxiety and control. Based on this discussion I suggest that the hesitancy expressed by donors about the information they are offered can be viewed as a form of resistance to an imposed sense of responsibility. Though the latter interpretation does allow us to appreciate the lack of interest in specified information, it still does not provide any feasible explanation as to why many donors nevertheless praise the idea of informed consent. To address this issue, I explore some of the meanings that can be ascribed to the donated tissue in relation to what Michel Foucault (1992) termed the 'practices of the self'. Blood can be imagined in different ways – as both an intimate part of the person and as a 'mere thing' – and this impreciseness is central to an understanding of informed consent procedures in biobank research.

Quiet medical examinations and talkative interviews

During their medical examinations at the public healthcare centres most participants also become donors and sign a consent form. The first informed consent form that was introduced in 1990 was called a 'donation act', and since then there have been different versions, each containing more information than the previous one. As mentioned above, however, few people pose any questions or pay particular attention to the information they are given. The nurses responsible for the examinations could partly confirm these observations. Before and after observing medical examinations I spoke to the nurse responsible, and I held focus group discussions with nurses at four of the five healthcare centres where I did interviews. Marilyn Strathern (1999) has commented that anthropology is the making of descriptions through the use of others' descriptions, and I consciously tried to relate the nurses' descriptions of their experiences of the examinations to my own with the hope of validating or challenging these. Some nurses claimed never to have had a question posed to them, not even from the ones who declined to donate. One nurse told me that: 'They've made up their minds before coming, they don't want to discuss [it]'. However, others reported that people have begun asking about the commercial use of the donated blood or expressing concern about their anonymity.

Even more surprising than the fact that the patients/donors asked the nurses relatively few questions, was that some nurses sought information from me. They wanted to know why the donors'/participants' social security number had to feature in the questionnaire that is submitted with the blood sample, what UmanGenomics was all about, and whether the company had access to all the tissue samples in the healthcare system. Some of them wanted to know because they had donated samples themselves and were apparently reminded of this by my research. However, not all the nurses seemed eager to ascertain for which purposes the samples would be used. One nurse had not heard about UmanGenomics nor had she read the consent form. Several nurses did not know about the right to withdraw consent on donated samples, which is a key piece of information according to the ethical review board that has approved the consent form. Others were very well-informed and highly alert to the new commercial uses of the biobank. One such nurse explained that she found the new and extended versions of the consent form an improvement because now she no longer felt that there were issues left unaddressed.[3] These nurses all described different forms of anxiety, but few of them expressed a concern to know more until they were confronted with the presence and queries of the anthropologist, then questions emerged concerning the blood they otherwise just collected as part of their daily work. Similarly, some concerns were articulated by the otherwise confident patients – who had also become biobank donors – when I asked them about the use of the blood samples that they had given.

Between anxiety and responsibility

Amongst the many different worries expressed in relation to genetics, eugenics and cloning were the most commonly voiced. Some of these came in response to a question I asked all participants: is there anything for which they would not like the researchers to use their blood sample? Usually this question was followed by a pause. One woman responded that: 'Research that has anything to do with cloning . . . I don't like that [. . .] Actually, that whole issue of looking into and manipulating the genes – It sounds . . . unhealthy to me.' When I asked whether she would accept gene therapy or attempts at 'manipulating' genes with the intention of curing illness, she immediately responded: 'Yes, of course, then it's alright!' She explained that she did not like research that simply wanted to 'normalize' everybody, which is how she perceived cloning and eugenics.

Another woman also saw 'manipulation of genes' as being related to cloning. In response to my question about uses of her blood that she would not accept, she said: 'I don't know. . . . Well, of course, it might be that they can clone – that somebody can do a copy of me? No [timid laugh] . . . I guess I haven't thought much about it . . . [but] I am a bit scared of this genetic manipulation.' I asked what she had in mind by the term 'genetic manipulation' and she said that she wasn't really sure. Several informants thought of genetic research as directly related to 'designer babies', and one woman explained that she supported research 'when it's about human suffering [. . .] or inherited defects, then it's okay. But to talk about for example homosexuality as an inherited defect? I'm not ready for that!' Her fear was that genetic research would be used for 'normalizing' people. In response to my question as to whether she thought it would be acceptable to 'normalize' schizophrenics with medicine based on genetic research, she was less certain.

One woman, diagnosed with depression, wondered whether, if geneticists had their way, she might not have been entitled to a life of her own. She had suffered from depression but she also felt that it had given her something: 'one wants to live without depressions, without the angst, but I also know that it has developed me – it has contributed . . . [There] is [a] sensitivity that follows in its wake.' The thought of research into the genetic component of a central aspect of her life felt offensive and potentially stigmatizing: 'modification' of some of her genes would approximate to the 'removal' of an aspect of her personhood. In response to my question, she also revealed that she did not know whether her donated blood sample would be used for genetic research; she had not read the consent form: 'no, I didn't read it, I just signed and left a sample'. She expected that it would contribute to new knowledge, to medical progress.

Thus, the aim of eradicating diseases by, for example, preventing the inheritance of certain genes from one generation to the next, can be perceived as amounting to the eradication of certain types of people. In this sense genes can be understood as being ascribed the attribute of personhood to the extent that some respondents saw that it amounted to genocide to attempt to screen for specific disease-related genes. There were other implicit references to eugenics: 'I'm scared if we end up in a situation where you'll only accept – let's say – elite-healthy people. That's what I'm scared of, that [. . .] you'll only want *perfect* people.' One woman said that it would be much better if research was focused on diseases rather than on genetic research, which she expected to deal with 'producing perfect babies'. Most such anxious responses contained only very vague formulations. Significantly, it was not the Biobank or the researchers associated with the university or UmanGenomics, but some undefined 'they' who were supposed to desire a certain kind of society of 'perfect babies' and 'elite-healthy people'. This resonates with the fact that the most common response to the question about the unacceptable uses of their donated blood was that patients/donors had simply never thought about it. Mostly, research – or at least the research they contributed to – was assumed to produce something benevolent.

The limited interest in the information provided in the consent forms is partly related to the informants having another purpose with regard to their attendance at the healthcare centre. They are there as patients to undergo medical examinations and so scrutinizing information about the Biobank would be a waste of time for them. But I believe there is something more to it than that. I suggest that it is also a way of addressing an implicit question of who should assume the responsibility for, on the one hand, potentially disastrous research and, on the other, the rejection of potentially benevolent research. Scientific research is inherently ambiguous, and this ambiguity might be pivotal to the success of informed consent.

The mixture of hopes and fears produced by so-called 'gene-talk' (Keller 2000) has been described by Paul Rabinow (1999) as creating an almost purgatorial atmosphere. An essential feature of this genetic purgatory is an overwhelming sense of responsibility. Around genetic technologies are generated images and expectations of a new world in which humankind is seen to have greater control over life itself. Possibly, many genetic technologies will fail (cf. Keller 2000), but the very intention of genetic research is to create and control aspects of human life until now beyond the reach of human intervention. Who should have responsibility for this kind of power? This question, implied in all of the promises, creates an intangible 'cloud of responsibility'.

Dominant Western traditions in moral philosophy relate responsibility to a common sense notion of causation: it is asserted that one attains responsibility for something if one caused it (Løgstrup 1996). The peculiar aspect of this tradition is the accentuation of personal responsibility: individuals presumably have intentions, which make them responsible for the consequences caused by their actions (Taylor 1985). Anthropological studies in comparative ethics have shown that the emphasis given to the individual in questions of responsibility and causation is not universal (Read 1955, Jackson 1982, 1998).[4] The search for a moral subject has also been challenged within science and technology studies. For example Catherine Waldby's (2000) re-reading of Martin Heidegger's seminal essay, 'The question concerning technology', outlines the limitations of a notion of causation that seeks to identify human beings as the causing agents and technologies simply as tools in their hands: 'Modern "technics" [. . .] is never simply at the disposal of "Man", but sets Man up and replaces and displaces him in dynamic ways' (Waldby 2000: 42). In other words, technologies have an efficacy of their own.

Can this complexity of causation be detected in my informants' diffuse perception of danger? And if the counter charge to danger is an urge for control, what, then, is presented as 'control'? I wish to suggest that informed consent procedures imply a search for an accountable moral subject while side-stepping the weight of moral responsibility by allowing this responsibility to be diffusely distributed. Informed consent has the double effect of both placing individuals in a position in which they have to make choices and freeing them from responsibility for the negative implications of the research to which they have consented by constructing a diffuse arrangement of donors who can be only semi-accountable agents. This network of agents is linked by a notion of public oversight, as I go on to argue below.

Some informants seem to insist on being given information, although they do not use this information in their decision-making. It appears to *feel right* to be given a choice, without the implications of that choice necessarily being considered in depth (cf. Rose 1999). This could be important to the workings of informed consent procedures. Furthermore, claiming the right to decide on the use of one's blood might be part of presenting oneself as a responsible person. It would thus reflect a certain ethics in the Foucauldian sense of practices of the self (Foucault 1983, 1992). In this case, informed consent procedures offer an opportunity of doing a certain work on oneself, the work of perceiving oneself as an autonomous responsible actor. The act of signing a consent sheet may then be one of numerous insignificant institutionally mediated practices through which individuals may experience themselves as being in control and being responsible – not for science but for themselves.

While informed consent might be valued as giving individuals a sense of control over and responsibility for *themselves*, informants talked about the public authorities as playing an important role in controlling *science*. UmanGenomics was launched with the public announcement that the county council and the state-owned University of Umeå would own more than 50 per cent of its shares. During spring 2002, the principle of majority ownership was abandoned as part of making UmanGenomics appear more attractive to investors. The renegotiation gave rise to some controversy, not least because public majority ownership had featured in the ethics policy and subsequently been included in the improved consent form (for an introduction to the controversy see Lövtrup 2003 or Hoeyer 2003a). Rather than engaging with the question of ownership per se, I would like to draw attention to the idiom in which public ownership has been discussed: it has been said to ensure public control through 'public oversight'. As I show below, the very concepts of control and oversight are used interchangeably by many informants.

Public oversight as collective and individual control

To understand the meanings attached to public 'oversight' (the Swedish word means to see into) we need to consider features of the ethnographic context not usually included in studies of informed consent.[5] The idea that public authorities can exercise control over science reflects a certain historical experience of state power in Sweden. The Swedish welfare state has an impressive record for ensuring economic growth, health benefits and housing improvements. The driving force over the 50-year period of 1870–1920, in which Sweden developed from one of Europe's poorest countries to one of its richest, is usually seen to be the popular movements which had – and still have – their stronghold in northern Sweden (Frykman and Löfgren 1987, Gustavsson 1991).[6] These popular movements drew on a particular Nordic enlightenment tradition that emphasized the importance of striving for knowledge as means of attaining the fruits of the future (Sørensen and Stråth 1997). In many Western societies, knowledge is talked of in spatial and visual metaphors (Lakoff and Johnson 1980, Salmond 1982) and there is a strong conflation of knowledge and control: to see is to know, and to know is to control. I suggest that what is extraordinary in northern Sweden is not only the degree to which these notions of vision, knowledge and control are fused, but that the vision, knowledge and control of the state is seen also to be that of the individual. Therefore, public ownership of UmanGenomics is seen as a way of ensuring state control and, as a consequence, individuals' control over the company's activities.

The conflation of state and individual control was evident throughout my fieldwork interviews with staff at the Biobank, donors, nurses and other informants. Rather than providing a range of examples of the ways in which the metaphors were articulated, I wish to point out how people objected when in the later part of my fieldwork I began mentioning that it was, after all, just metaphors. Mostly, informants defended the substance of the claim that majority ownership would constitute actual control with reference to the Swedish system of public records (*offentlighetsprincipen*). In principle, all public documents are open to everyone and this means, I was repeatedly told, that all individuals in Swedish society share the oversight of the state. If something was publicly owned then individuals would be in a position to know what was going on too, and in this way they really were in control. However, knowledge of risks is not necessarily the same as controlling risks. I would suggest that just because county representatives have access to see the activities of UmanGenomics, it does not mean that they understand all aspects of these activities and their social, ethical or scientific implications. Certainly, the vaguely articulated anxieties about genetic research, which are discussed above, are in no sense under control simply because county officials sit on the board. All technologies can be considered inherently ambiguous (Jackson 2002b), and the same technology that offers cures for diseases might equally be involved in those aspects of research about which some of my informants expressed concern.

However, it should be acknowledged that the Swedish system of public records is very impressive. There is a real set of experiences of the state behind the argument that state knowledge is practically the same as individual knowledge. Public trust in the state is supported by legal and institutional arrangements, which were highly regarded by many (but not all) donors, nurses, academic researchers and staff at UmanGenomics, who invoked an image of Swedish law – and what was loosely referred to as Swedish 'rules' – as providing safeguards beyond question. On the governance of biobanks, Sweden has passed a law that also emphasizes informed consent, public oversight through research ethics committees and security of personal data (Socialdepartementet 2002). This legislation, like the ethics policy of Uman-Genomics, is principally concerned with public oversight and the information given to donors, rather than with issues of how such data are then subsequently used by whom and for what purposes. Although it also specifies how tissue should be stored, for example, it does not address the issues articulated by my informants as sources of anxiety. Nevertheless, the fact that there is a law is viewed by some as indication of public control.

Another notable aspect of this discussion about public oversight is the cultural specificity of northern Sweden. This is an area that is characterized by small dispersed settlements, which sustain strong local networks. This, I would claim, reinforces further the experience of public control. Everybody more or less knows everybody.[7] An employee at UmanGenomics related to me that it was important the company was based locally because people would know that employees would not dare to do anything strange: if they did they would be socially castigated. He told me that: 'I've got to be able to show my face in town, you know'.

While the triad of vision, knowledge and control may be bound up with the creation of institutional safeguards, such as the majority stake in Uman-Genomics, it does not eliminate totally the sense of uncertainty. In spite of the trust expressed in the conflation of the state and individual oversight, public authorities are not immune to criticism. On the contrary, there has been an intense tradition within Sweden of criticizing the state, particularly for its misuse of power. Lately, such criticism has contributed much to the modification of the welfare state towards what Nikolas Rose (1999) has called the 'facilitating' state, the primary task of which is to offer choices to citizens rather than the provision of universal services. The introduction of informed consent procedures into new domains of decision-making such as donation to biobanks can be seen as part of this trend. Rather than making decisions, the state ensures individuals have access to information and allows them to make choices. But how do the procedures of informed consent carried out in the healthcare centres relate to the anxieties expressed by my informants and in what ways do these offer them any control over the research done on their donated tissue?

Informed consent as a means of control?

Donors rarely mentioned an explicit personal responsibility for the potentially negative implications of genetic research. Instead, most informants talked about a responsibility for helping science to alleviate illness and pain. As with their fears, some had very abstract hopes. Others referred to diseased children in their family for whom they wished a cure. Their involvement in research seems embedded in what Carlos Novas (2001) has termed the 'political economy of hope' or what I call the historical narrative of progress. This narrative is connected with the history of the Swedish welfare state, which has continued to prosper throughout the greater part of the twentieth century. One informant related that if I had lived to see, as he had, poor people with inadequate water supply, poor infrastructure, no heating and low education move into proper houses and develop to master good jobs, I would learn to appreciate progress. Narratives of progress, just like confidence in public oversight, reflect some very real historical experiences. However, following the events of the twentieth century, it is 'safe' to say that so does the fear that technologies may be used for something far less benevolent. Informants are familiar with narratives of both hope and fear, but which one of these different available narratives informs their choice in the actual situation where they decide whether or not to donate a sample for future research? What does informed consent offer to individuals who hope for the benefits of genetic research while also wishing to exercise some control over it to avoid the dangers they fear?

Following Michael Jackson (2002a, 2002b) we might suggest that their situation is one that is characterized by having to make a moral judgement. Jackson describes moral judgement as a way of dealing with matters that are beyond the direct influence or control of individuals. When a technology is judged good or evil it acquires a place in our conceptual universe and is less troublesome, so to speak, as Jackson remarks: 'to deliver a judgement is to close a case' (Jackson 2002a: 143). Jackson further contends that when people feel that they are in control of technologies they are much more likely to deem them benevolent and vice versa. The narrative of progress entails a discourse of empowerment and greater control through technology. People in Västerbotten generally hold strong beliefs in the benefits of science. By contrast, people in Tonga strongly opposed an Australia-based biotech company's proposals to establish a genetic database on the people of the tiny South Pacific nation (Inter Press Service 2002). Jackson (2002a) argues that the historical experience of technologies indicates whether they will in the final analysis be to the benefit of people such as the Tongans or exported to more affluent nations. Seen in relation to the very diverse responses in Västerbotten and Tonga, this might begin to tell us something about why some communities tend to choose a narrative of hope and others one of fear when enrolled in biotech adventures.

There is another aspect to the issue of control. Drawing on American pragmatism Susan Whyte (1997, 1999) has shown that there is a inclination among Ugandans at the risk of AIDS to opt for the *security* of family networks, rather than the *certainty* of knowing their HIV status. In contrast, my Swedish informants value certainty very highly. In relation to disease a clear majority even talk of a sense of duty to know about risks, which is exemplified by their attendance at the medical examinations that provide them with a risk profile. However, when it comes to the informed consent procedure they are less apprehensive. Whereas knowledge about their cholesterol might make them change their diet – it leaves new options open – it is unclear exactly what information would make them change their mind as to donate or not. How will they know if a research project on cardiovascular diseases will advance methods which can subsequently be used for purposes they dislike? Here the notion of certainty becomes very opaque. If donors prefer the tacit sense of security expressed in a trust relationship with a nurse in the medical examination rather than to discuss openly about what will be done with their donated blood sample, it is perhaps not so surprising.

The interview as an extended informed consent

Having signed the consent form, donors do not have to think more about it: the case is settled until an anthropologist arrives asking questions about their attitudes to the developments in the biosciences. An interview has similarities to the informed consent procedure, but is prolonged in the sense that it obliges donors to adopt a more active stance: during an interview you have to talk back, you cannot simply sign the form and get on. In line with Jackson's argument, we might say that I changed the informants' relationship to the technologies with my questions. Without my questioning the informants may have felt in a position of control, to be free to help research, to be the benevolent provider of a gift. However, my questions are new to them and clearly touch upon unfamiliar issues. They are now in a position of being confronted with something about which they feel very little control and, as a consequence, become less positive towards research. In agreement with Jackson we might say that their perception of research technologies reflects their sense of power in relation to these technologies. As long as the donors are with the nurse, the medical technologies are primarily tools at their disposal, but when future applications of science are discussed with the anthropologist, donors are less certain about who will benefit.

The examples of anxiety provided above are both very real and very abstract. Do they belong to the specific situation? Are the informants really faced with a 'risk' that can be assessed in relation to the specific blood sample? Gerda Reith (2002) amongst others wants us to reconsider Ulrich Beck's (1997) hypothesis that today we are surrounded by *more* risk. Instead, Reith argues that risk has become a way of perceiving and dealing with things that creates notions of responsibility as described above. The pronounced anxiety that I have reported on from my interviews could be seen in this perspective as an expression not of more risk but of more knowledge of things that may go wrong. If we momentarily accept this premise,[8] informed consent procedures then shift from being simply a device for handling risk or anxiety to *a site for the production of risk*: here people are confronted with knowledge that may potentially create anxiety. The same could of course be said of my interviews. The interviews were not simple channels through which anxiety was conveyed; they were sites for the production of certain types of reflections.

With their prolonged character the interviews might have given a view on the possible effect of emphasizing informed consent in this type of research, namely increased awareness of anxieties and the accompanying responsibility.

The common response of not paying too much attention to the information in the informed consent form may then be seen as a kind of resistance – one of the mundane tacit practices of opposition described by Michel de Certeau (1988) – to greater knowledge, to greater risk and the sense of responsibility that would be conferred on people simply trying to do their duty by contributing 20 millilitres of blood. By not reading the consent form people quietly resist what Judith Green (1997) has termed a privatized risk management. However, the anthropological interview (re)imposes the obligation on donors to make a personal risk assessment. The interview induces moral choices on the informants, in which they settle complex issues by judging them good or bad. Might informed consent procedures make an implicit move towards such effects? If so, informed consent becomes moral in a different way than that implied by the ethics policy adopted by UmanGenomics, where it was supposed to be a means for ensuring the dignity of individuals through the execution of their rational autonomy. The informed consent becomes moral because it creates a sense of obligation to take a stance. Our philosophical heritage would expect us to relate the moral choice to assessments of causation and consequences of science – the personal responsibility for what we bring about. But, as shown above, people do not try to ascertain what types of project they contribute to. Therefore, I argue that the moral choice they make hinges on something else that can be understood through notions of personhood.

The spirit in the blood: protecting themselves as agents

Individuals who chose not to donate to the Biobank rarely gave an explanation that has anything to do with the specific aspects of the proposed research. Indeed, several even said that UmanGenomics sounded like an excellent idea, and thought genetic research could be very beneficial. Reasons for refusal had little to do with assessments of social or individual risk, but were more related to the specific situation, their perception of the medical examination and a reluctance to let other objectives interfere with their personal health check. As one person said: 'I do this [medical examination] for myself'. Though neither donors nor people refusing to donate paid any particular attention to the information provided in the consent form, many felt that informed consent was important to them. The solution to this paradox – of wanting something which apparently they did not use for anything – could be found in the ambiguous meanings it is possible to ascribe to the donated tissue.

Several informants talked about the blood as *part of* themselves. One woman even said: 'It is part of me . . . my blood, it really *is* me, straight up'.[9] In discussions with informants outside the clinic I similarly encountered very strong personal associations with blood. One informant conceived that there was no difference between him and his blood because the blood (or rather the genes in blood) at any time could be used for generating another him. Here images of cloning impinge on conceptions of what constitutes a person's essence. One exchange during an interview at a healthcare centre was particularly telling on this issue:

Informant:	Well, this thing . . . what's it called [pause] gene − . . . mutations, or what's the name? When they make copies?
Anthropologist:	Cloning?
Informant:	Yes − You want to skip that!
Anthropologist:	[pause] What is it that you find wrong with cloning?
Informant:	Pardon?
Anthropologist:	They won't make any clones using your blood, don't get me wrong, I just thought − what is it that's wrong with cloning − why do you think it is wrong?
Informant:	Well, I think that *everybody* has a right to be . . . their own . . . person.

Implicitly, this informant found that the person and the genes are one and the same. Similarly, I described earlier how genes were sometimes seen as integral parts of the donating person when eradication of genes linked with certain conditions was discussed. If genes were eradicated, so would these persons. This type of reasoning indicates that genes can be conceived as the very essence of the person. A test tube of blood thus lends itself to imagination as a container of personhood and becomes an object of the moral rights and duties attributed to living persons, including the right to live and the right to make choices.

However, the imaginary is not always so, and it may differ from person to person and from time to time. The informant I mentioned above who held that there was a very strong association between his sense of personhood and blood was a molecular biologist. When he was working with blood samples that were anonymous and encountered in test tubes, they could become de-personalized, thus lose their potential for 'personhood'.[10] Clearly, then blood can be the focus of multiple interpretations even by the same person. Similarly, a nurse told me that she had taken the samples for years and never thought about it until I came along. 'Blood is just blood' had been her attitude, but now she said that she realized its importance: 'It is part of the person donating it.' My work added to the meanings she attributed to blood.

In my own fieldwork I had also moved between different understandings of blood. Once I was shown around the storage facilities at the Medical Biobank. We had been walking down the rows of freezers and had seen the orderly storage principles, and had been told about the security arrangements surrounding the tissue collection. The room was as calm as my mood: I took notes, looked down at individual blood samples, and noted that each line in a rack came from one person. As my guide and I went out the door and turned off the light, he mentioned, 'So this is where we keep the blood of 85,000 people'. His words conjured up an image in my mind and I felt that I had visited a kind of graveyard or a sanctuary in which 85,000 people were kept. I reflect on this incident here because it is a way of showing how the actual tissue, the millilitres of blood, stored in the Biobank are open for many interpretations: they do not hold one specific meaning; they are both human and non-human, both living persons and dead objects. In this light, the paradoxical behaviour of people on the one hand requesting a choice and on the other not showing interest in the information expected to inform that choice makes sense. People can easily dispense with a sample because it is 'only blood', and then in a subsequent research interview feel concerned about the blood being used for purposes they dislike because the interview reconnects them, their sense of personhood, to that sample again.

Robert Desjarlais (2000) has argued that institutional arrangements permeated by power inequalities facilitate different experiences of self and particular constructions of personhood. He defines personhood in the sense that I have used the concept here as 'the state of being a socially recognized and engaged human being, acknowledged by law as the subject of rights and duties, with a distinct character or "personae"' though adding abilities which can hardly be ascribed to blood, namely 'the bearer of faculties of communication, reason, and moral judgment' (Desjarlais 2000: 478). Like Green (1997) who investigated the procedures that create privatized risk management, Desjarlais suggests that governmental arrangements, of which informed consent procedures are an example, shape perceptions of personhood, including ideas about what it takes to present one self as a responsible actor. I depart from Desjarlais in his implicit top-down assumption. Rather than seeing personhood as shaped *by* a governmental policy, I suggest that certain perceptions of personhood emerge *through* these policies and thus facilitate particular governmental possibilities. The practices of self are part of creating a pressure for more choices – part of facilitating an understanding of informed choice as a 'solution' to a problem of control.

Different issues become the focus of moral concern and subsequent governmental arrangements at different times (cf. Foucault 1994). Anne Kerr (2004) has suggested that the continuities between past and present in governmental techniques should be recognized when understanding how a new research technology such as biobanks is being handled (cf. Koch 2002). She talks of notions of 'genetic citizenship' (not personhood) and opposes the suggestion that citizenship is radically changed just because we see different articulations of it. Similarly, I contend that we might find that the practices of self are not radically changed just because 20 millilitres of blood has become the object of new negotiations about personhood. Desjarlais adds that different notions of personhood may be at work simultaneously. The latter point departs from the ways in which much scholarship has discussed the concept of person in broad terms as Western/non-Western notions (Read 1955, Mauss 1986, Hollos and Leis 2002). I would argue that an awareness of such diversity seems suitable for an understanding of recent and sporadic arrangements such as informed consent for tissue-based genetic research.

When paying limited attention to the actual information about research purposes, people are not 'irrationally' dismissing the information they need to assess the research to which they are contributing. Their decision to contribute and the feelings that this invokes can just as easily relate to the sociocultural context in which they live and their perception of the relationship between themselves (momentarily represented by 20 millilitres of blood) and the authorities and company asking for access to this aspect of their person. Information about the research agenda would be of little importance, since it can hardly help them to assess whether their blood will be used for research with implications they may oppose. The use of informed consent is different in relation to biobank research compared with clinical trials, where research participants assess a risk incurred on their living body. With biobank research they assess what type of research they want to support without the actual research projects having any influence on their health. Therefore, informed consent plays a different role in introducing a sense of responsibility, producing and controlling anxiety, re-connecting the blood and the donor.

Conclusion

Biobanks are sites for genetic research that amplify an ambivalence that has always surrounded medicine: it is the power to enact life and death decisions. The abstract and diffuse dangers and the intangible responsibility related to potentially negative social developments of this research are responded to with a set of organizational procedures and discourses emphasizing individual choice and personal freedom. Even measures presented as providing some degree of public oversight are basically a matter of the state ensuring the individual access to information and choice.

I have suggested reinterpreting informed consent procedures in various ways: they might be doing several things at once, and serve different functions for different people and institutions. It *both* protects the agent's autonomy and integrity (as many proponents of informed consent claim) *and* produces autonomous actors. It *both* reflects a respect for people's interest in knowing what happens to their blood *and* creates that interest by making them think of their blood as part of themselves. It *both* provides a sense of control through the offered choice *and* produces anxiety because the choice confronts the potential donor with an intangible responsibility. Likewise the donated blood can be imagined as *both* dead tissue *and* as integral to the donor's agency.

The ambiguous status of the donated tissue might have further implications for future discussions about attitudes towards the commercialization of biobanks. It appears that there is a tendency for a strong aversion to commercialization when blood is conceived as part of the person. On the other hand, when it is conceived of as an object, as a resource, people seem ready to discuss whether this resource can help attract inward investment to this rather marginalized region in Sweden. The controversy during spring 2002 mentioned above about the ownership of UmanGenomics has led to a number of public accusations that may have impaired the image of private companies in this domain. I have interviewed nurses who reported that donation rates have gone down, but I have not as yet sufficient documentation of this. It would be interesting to see whether the doubt introduced by these accusations sustains a personalization of the stored blood so that the trust relationship between the authorities in charge of the biobank and the donor becomes conceptualized in terms of what is done to the stored 'person'.

Informed consent procedures address societal problems and existential anxieties through a philosophical tradition that emphasizes personal choice. The point of the procedures is ostensibly to allow choices to be given to 'persons' who may view themselves as 'causing agents' of positive effects. Thanks to a history of progress, a conceptualization of control as relying on vision and knowledge and a conflation of the state and individual, the donating subjects may see themselves as contributing to an economy of hope. Donors can hardly view themselves as 'causing' potentially negative effects. Rather, they are protecting their sense of themselves as agents. Informed consent procedures may further stimulate a sense of responsibility for contributing to benevolent research because there will be no research if there is no research material, but these procedures simultaneously allow a diffuse arrangement of responsibility for the intangible negative implications, matching the diffuse perception of danger reported by my informants. This might be central to the recent success of informed consent procedures in the governance of biobanks. The two levels of danger that this chapter has addressed – on the one hand the individual level of everyday life in which science and technology form part of a narrative of progress and on the other the societal level where humankind is now in a position to both 'duplicate' and destroy itself – become conflated when informed consent procedures are introduced as decision-making regimes in relation to biobank research. The ambiguity not only of what is donated to the biobank, but also of the informed consent procedure through which it is handed over, is perhaps more significant and more potent than we readily acknowledge.

Acknowledgements

An earlier version of this paper was presented at the EASA Conference in Copenhagen August 2002, in a panel convened by Gislí Pálsson and Sarah Franklin. I would like to thank the people attending the session for their useful comments. I would also like to thank Lene Koch, Richard Tutton and Oonagh

Corrigan for insightful criticism at later stages of the paper's transformation into the present chapter. The Ethics in Healthcare Programme in Sweden has generously supported the fieldwork (grant no. 2000/56) together with the Nordic Committee for Social Science Research (NOS-S).

Notes

1. This chapter is based on 10 months of anthropological fieldwork carried out intermittently between June 2000 and March 2003. Most time was spent in and around Umeå, though two locations in Lapland were also visited.

2. Informed consent procedures and the ethical review boards are intertwined because the main task of the boards is to assess the adequacy of the information presented to potential donors (see also Greely 1998, Eriksson 2001).

3. The first consent form, the 'donation act', basically stated that the blood was donated for future research purposes. In later versions the type of diseases that will be researched, the name of the company and other specifications have been added.

4. Also, the notion of intentionality has been critiqued for relying on false instrumentality (Myhre 1998).

5. Exceptions do exist, notably Gordon and Paci (1997). Tutton (2002) has also shown how local histories influence people's perception of not only the research in question, but the benefit they might expect from their participation.

6. In particular the temperance movement, the workers' movement and the free churches. Self-discipline was pivotal to all three movements and it was combined with praise of solidarity and confidence in science as a tool for conquering the future (Qvarsell 1986, Ambjörnsson 1988). For a more elaborate discussion of this element of the history of the welfare state in relation to the current informed consent procedures, see Hoeyer (2003b).

7. Umeå is for northern Swedish standards a very impressive town with 105,006 inhabitants. Nevertheless, within professional groups most people know one another even in Umeå. Västerbotten County as a whole has 254,818 inhabitants dispersed over 59,194 km^2 (figures from Västerbotten County 31 December 2001).

8. It is a premise that can be disputed, and often is. It can easily be argued that the potential high-tech dangers of our times are more devastating than ever before, a nuclear war being one example (Kemp 1991). Such dangers, however, are only faintly related to individual research projects and even less to the everyday lives of my informants, who employ a narrative of progress when praising the decrease of dangers in their everyday lives.

9. Not everybody associated so strongly with their blood. For a discussion of this, see Hoeyer (2002).

10. I have discussed the role of the ethical model of UmanGenomics in depersonalizing the blood elsewhere, see Hoeyer (2002).

References

Abbott, S. (1999). 'Sweden sets ethical standards for use of genetic "biobanks"', *Nature* 400: 3.

Ambjörnsson, R. (1988). *Den skötsamme arbetaren. Idéer och ideal i ett norrländskt sågverkssamhälle 1880–1930*, Malmö: Carlsson Bokförlag.

Beck, U. (1997). *Risikosamfundet. På vej mod en ny modernitet*, Copenhagen: Hans Reitzels Forlag.

Beskow, L.M., Burke, W., Merz, J.F. *et al.* (2001). 'Informed consent for population-based research involving genetics', *Journal of the American Medical Association* 286: 2315–2321.

de Certeau, M. (1988). *The Practice of Everyday Life*, London: University of California Press.

Desjarlais, R. (2000). 'The makings of personhood in a shelter for people considered homeless and mentally ill', *Ethos* 27: 466–489.

Eriksson, S. (2001). 'Informed consent and biobanks', in M. Hansson (ed.) *The Use of Human Biobanks: Ethical, Social, Economical and Legal Aspects*, Uppsala: Universitets-tryckeriet.

Foucault, M. (1983). 'On the genealogy of ethics: An overview of work in progress', in H.L. Dreyfus and P. Rabinow (eds) *Michel Foucault. Beyond Structuralism and Hermeneutics*, Chicago: University of Chicago Press.

Foucault, M. (1992). *The Use of Pleasure. The History of Sexuality: 2*, London: Penguin Books.

Foucault, M. (1994). *Viljen til viden, seksualitetens historie vol. 1* [The Will to Power], Copenhagen: Det Lille Forlag.

Frykman, J. and Löfgren, O. (1987). *Culture Builders. A Historical Anthropology of Middle-Class Life*, London: Rutgers UP.

Gordon, D.R. and Paci, E. (1997). 'Disclosure practices and cultural narratives: understanding concealment in silence around cancer in Tuscany, Italy', *Social Science and Medicine* 44: 1433–1452.

Greely, H. (1998). 'Legal, ethical and social issues in human genome research', *Annual Review of Anthropology* 27: 473–503.

Green, J. (1997). 'Risk and high modernity', in *Risk and Misfortune. A Social Construction of Accidents*, London: UCL Press.

Gustavsson, A. (1991). 'Vanan, synden och världen i väckelsemiljöer. Om tron och vardagslivets ordning', in J. Frykman and O. Löfgren (eds) *Svenska vanor och ovanor*, Stockholm: Natur och Kultur.

Hallgren, C.G. (1994). *Västerbottensprojektet 1992–93 och FoB 90 del 1 och 2*, Umeå, Sweden: Västerbottens Läns Landstings Samhällsmedicinska Enhet.

Hallgren, C.G. (1995). *Västerbottensprojektet 1992–93 och FoB 90 del 3 och 4*, Umeå, Sweden: Västerbottens Läns Landstings Samhällsmedicinska Enhet.

Hoeyer, K. (2002). 'Conflicting notions of personhood in genetic research', *Anthropology Today* 18: 9–13.

Hoeyer, K. (2003a). Personhood in commercial genetic research. Some notes on commodification. Paper presented at ASA Decennial Conference, University of Manchester, 14–18 July.

Hoeyer, K. (2003b). '"Science is really needed – that's all I know": Informed consent and the non-verbal practices of collecting blood for genetic research in Sweden', *New Genetics and Society* 22(3): 198–212.

Hollos, M. and Leis, P. (2002). 'Remodeling concepts of the self: an Ijo example', *Ethos* 29: 371–387.

Inter Press Service (2002). 'Opposition stalls genetic profiling: plan for Tonga', published 18 February 2002, downloaded 31 June 2002 at www.hi.is.

Jackson, M. (1982). *Allegories of the Wilderness. Ethics and Ambiguity in Kuranko Narratives*, Bloomington: Indiana University Press.

Jackson, M. (1998). *Minima Ethographica. Intersubjectivity and Anthropological Project*, London: University of Chicago Press.

Jackson, M. (2002a). 'Biotechnology and the critique of globalisation', *Ethnos* 67: 141–154.

Jackson, M. (2002b). 'Familiar and foreign bodies: a phenomenological exploration of the human–technology interface', *Journal of the Royal Anthropological Institute* 8: 333–346.

Keller, E.F. (2000). *The Century of the Gene*, London: Harvard University Press.

Kemp, P. (1991). *Det uerstattelige. En teknologi-etik*, Copenhagen: Spektrum.

Kerr, A. (2004). 'Genetics and citizenship: Exploring transformations', draft to be published in N. Ster (ed.) *Biotechnology Between Commerce and Civil Society*, London: Transaction Publishers.

Koch, L. (2002). 'The government of genetic knowledge', in S. Lundin and L. Åkesson (eds) *Gene Technology and Economy*, Lund: Nordic Academic Press.

Lakoff, G. and Johnson, M. (1980). *Metaphors We Live By*, London: The University of Chicago Press.

Løgstrup, K.E. (1996 [1971]). *Etiske begreber og problemer*, Copenhagen: Gyldendal.

Lövtrup, M. (2003). 'Drömmen om bioklippet slutade i affärsmässig anemi', *Dagens Medicin*, May 26–27.

Mauss, M. (1986 [1938]). 'A category of the human mind: The notion of person person; the notion of self', trans. by W.D. Halls, in M. Carrithers, A. Collins and S. Lukes (eds) *The Category of the Human Person. Anthropology, Philosophy, History*, Cambridge: Cambridge University Press.

Merz, J.F., McGee, G.E. and Sankar, P. (2004). '"Iceland Inc."?: On the ethics of commercial population genomics', *Social Science and Medicine* 58(6): 1201–1209.

Myhre, K.C. (1998). 'The anthropological concept of action and its problem: a new approach based on Marcel Mauss and Aristotle', *Journal of the Anthropological Society of Oxford* 29: 121–134.

Nilsson, A. and Rose, J. (1999). 'Sweden takes steps to protect tissue banks', *Science* 286: 894.

Novas, C. (2001). 'The political economy of hope: the labour of expecting cures'. Paper presented at the PFGS Colloquium 5, 20–21 June, University of Nottingham.

Qvarsell, R. (1986). 'Indledning', *Framtidens tjänst. Ur folkemmets idéhistoria*, Malmö: Gidlunds.

Rabinow, P. (1999). *French DNA. Trouble in purgatory*, London: University of Chicago Press.

Read, K.E. (1955). 'Morality and the concept of the person among the Gahuku-Gama', *Oceania* 25: 233–282.

Reith, G. (1999). 'The idea of chance', in *The Age of Change*, London: Routledge.

Rose, N. (1999). *Powers of Freedom. Reframing Political Thought*, Cambridge: Cambridge University Press.

Salmond, A. (1982). 'Theoretical landscapes', in D. Parkin (ed.) *Semantic Anthropology*, London: Academic Press.

Socialdepartementet (2002). Lag om Biobanker i Hälso- och Sjukvården m.m. [Law on Biobanks in Public Healthcare]. (2002: 297).

Sørensen, Ø. and Stråth, B. (eds) (1997). *The Cultural Construction of Norden*, Oslo: Scandinavian University Press.

Strathern, M. (1999). *Property, Substance and Effect. Anthropological Essays on Persons and Things*, London: The Athlone Press.

Taylor, C. (1985). 'The person', in M. Carrithers, A. Collins and S. Lukes (eds) *The Category of the Human Person. Anthropology, Philosophy, History*, Cambridge: Cambridge University Press.

Tutton, R. (2002). '"Gift relationships" in genetic research', *Science as Culture* 11: 524–542.

Västerbottensprojektet (1991). *Livsmedelsmärkning i Norsjö Kommun*, Umeå, Sweden: Umeå Universitet.

Waldby, C. (2000). *The Visible Human Project. Informatic Bodies and Posthuman Medicine*, London: Routledge.

Whyte, S. (1997). *Questioning Misfortune. The Pragmatics of Uncertainty in Eastern Uganda*, Cambridge: Cambridge University Press.

Whyte, S. (1999). 'Pragmatisme. Akademisk og anvendt', *Tidskriftet Antropologi* 40: 129–140.

Chapter 7

Abandoning informed consent

The case of genetic research in population collections

Jane Kaye

Introduction

The term 'population collection' started to emerge as a concept at the beginning of 2000 to describe the growing number of proposals for establishing genetic databases that were being announced around the world. It is a term that is suggestive of the type of research to be carried out – population genetics – but also describes a significant characteristic of such databases.[1] Population collections, unlike other medical research databases, will contain the personal medical information and DNA samples from individuals of a whole population. This population can include a whole country, such as Estonia, Iceland and Singapore, or a regional group such as the Västerbotten region of Sweden and Newfoundland in Canada. As discussed elsewhere in this volume, the purpose of pooling these primary sources of information is to provide a repository of information that can be used as a research tool, primarily to investigate the interactions between genes, environment and lifestyle that are thought to be responsible for common diseases. Information within the population collection can be kept for many years and used for multiple, secondary research purposes, by different researchers simultaneously. In the case of Iceland and Estonia, access by third parties is based on a fee with the intention that the population collections will be self-financing. Private companies will establish many of the population collections, with the exception of the Estonian and Singaporean proposals.

The proposal to establish the Icelandic Health Sector Database, the world's first population collection, was met with international and domestic condemnation. The main objection to the Icelandic population collection was that informed consent, the internationally agreed standard for biomedical research, was not sought. Instead, Icelandic citizens were only given the possibility of 'opting out' of the Health Sector Database. This 'opt-out' applied to both the collation of information from different sources in the population collection and for the secondary research use of the information in the population collection. The Icelandic authorities relied on the public interest exemption that is permitted under Directive 95/46/EC on the Protection of Individuals with Regard to Automatic Processing of Personal Data,[2] which has been developed in accordance with principles of medical research practice. The Directive stipulates common standards across the EU for the protection of individual privacy when data are 'processed'. European and national laws on data processing apply generally to the use of genetic data.

In this chapter I will argue that it is not possible to apply the principle of informed consent to the new context of population collections, but neither should the exceptions to informed consent, which have been allowed for medical research on the basis of the public interest, be used. I will discuss some of the issues around the use of genetic information in population collections and make some suggestions as to the protections that should be offered to individuals if informed consent cannot be obtained.

The requirements of consent

Consent is the threshold requirement for the use of identifiable medical data in medical research practice and the privacy law of the European Union. The requirement of consent is based on the principle of autonomy, and that 'respect for agents and persons requires that nothing be done to them without their consent' (O'Neill 2001: 691). Within the medical context consent is essential to research practice and the decision not to obtain consent for research that has no therapeutic benefit for the individual cannot be taken lightly. According to Alexander Capron (1991) consent acts as a reminder that autonomy must be considered, it improves research by developing good research design and it has a normalizing effect on the relationship between the researcher and the subject. However, within data protection law and in medical research the standard of consent differs. In medical research the threshold standard is informed consent, whereas Directive 95/46/EC requires explicit consent for the use of medical information. Both of these consent models require that individuals be given sufficient information on which to base a decision and therefore respect an individual's right to choose. One of the most controversial issues in the Icelandic debate was whether informed consent should be applied to the secondary use of medical information in the population collection. However, the very nature of population collections makes it very difficult to apply either of these different requirements of consent to population collections.

While it is generally acknowledged that informed consent is an established principle of medical research, it is also accepted that there are many different interpretations of what informed consent actually means and requires. The internationally agreed standard for medical research is informed consent as laid down in the World Medical Association's Declaration of Helsinki (2000). The principles of the Declaration are reiterated in the European Convention on Human Rights and Biomedicine 1997. The general principle is that this consent should be obtained prior to the collection of information and the commencement of the research. The Declaration states that:

In any research on human beings, each potential subject must be adequately informed of the aims, methods, anticipated benefits and potential hazards of the study and the discomfort that it may entail. He or she should be informed that he or she is at liberty to abstain from participation in the study and that he or she is free to withdraw his or her consent to participation at any time. The physician should then obtain the subjects' freely-given informed consent preferably in writing.

(World Medical Association 2000, para 22)

Informed consent respects individual autonomy, as involvement is dependent upon a voluntary, expressed consent based on information about the research proposal. Information must be provided to participants so they can make their own evaluation of the risks and benefits of research (see Corrigan chapter 5 this volume). This formulation was originally designed for single research projects within a medical setting, involving physical intervention. For this reason there is an emphasis on telling individuals about the potential hazards and any discomfort that the research may entail. It also stipulates this should be done before the research commences, so that an individual can make an informed decision about whether to be involved. In its formulation the requirements are not about informational harm or secondary research, but are more in line with traditional single research projects involving physical experimentation. In much of the ethical reasoning about the merits of research, harm is often considered in terms of physical risk rather than in terms of privacy, and this is evident in this formulation. The Declaration of Helsinki also states that the privacy of individuals should be respected, but this is not reflected in the informed consent provisions. For example, there is no provision to inform individuals how information will be used. It is with some difficulty that these requirements can be applied to population collections where the concern is with multiple research projects and where there is no physical discomfort involved in the medical research.

European Directive 95/46/EC requires that explicit consent is required for the processing of medical information. Individuals should be informed of the data processor, the type of data to be collected and from whom, details of the purposes of the data processing and to whom data will be communicated, and any rights of access or rectification (Directive 95/46/EC Art. 8,10,11). Unlike informed consent guidelines, the data protection legislation does not require that individuals should be informed of the risks and benefits of using the information. The closest the Directive 95/46/EC gets to imposing a positive duty to inform in this way, is by requiring that data processors inform individuals if they can withdraw their consent and the consequences involved. Instead the Directive requires that individuals should be provided with information about the data processing and then leaves it to the individual to assess the risks and benefits. The difference between the two different kinds of consent is that guidelines on informed consent are concerned with information regarding the broader research protocol, whereas the Directive is a lot narrower, being concerned only with the use of data and not the merits of the research in general.

Problems in applying consent

There are a number of problems in applying the requirements of informed and explicit consent to population collections. With reference to the inclusion of information in a collection, it is difficult to meet the requirements for information before research commences as required by informed and explicit consent provisions. This is because all of the research uses of the population collection cannot be anticipated when the data are first collected. This is due to the nature of population collections, which are large repositories of information that can be aggregated, linked, manipulated and continually added to over time. The fact that the data can be continually added to and kept for many years, means all the research questions and the researchers who may become involved cannot be anticipated at the time of the initial collection of the information. This makes it difficult to apply the requirements of informed consent and to supply individuals with specific information on each project, its aims, methods and researchers prior to information being collected. It is also difficult to inform individuals of the specific users of the data and the processing purposes as required by explicit consent. While it would be possible to do this in broad terms at the time of collection, it is not possible to be specific about the details of research that may be carried out in the future. Not being able to do this undermines the respect for autonomy that the consent measures are designed to protect, and the data protection legislation's requirement that individuals should be told of the research uses of their data prior to collection.

While it is not possible to inform individuals of all the research uses at the initial collection of information, it would also be difficult to gain further consent before the commencement of different secondary research. Once the population collection has started it is possible to know who the researchers are and the type of research that will be carried out on the data. However, at this stage it is difficult to obtain informed or explicit consent because of the impracticalities of contacting all the people who have information in a population collection. In Iceland, the Health Sector Database will contain information on 285,000 people, and the proposed Estonian Genome Project will have information on 1.5 million people. If the principles of informed consent were applied strictly it would mean that at the beginning of every new research project all the people in the population collection would have to be contacted. They would have to be informed of the aims, methods, sources of funding, any possible conflicts of interest, institutional affiliations of the researcher, the anticipated benefits and potential risks of the study and the discomfort it may entail. This would make a population collection unworkable, but may also unduly inconvenience participants if they had to consent to every enquiry that was made of the database. Informed consent would require an assessment of the benefits and risks of each type of research for each individual whereas this would not be the case for explicit consent. However, explicit consent would still require that individuals were informed of the details of the processing.

The requirements of informed and explicit consent also place a heavy emphasis on the individual, ignoring the way in which genetic information can illuminate the connections between family members. Janet Dolgin (2000) argues genetics creates a new concept of the family based on biology: 'The genetic family is defined through tests and diagnoses, developed as part of the new genetics' (Dolgin 2000: 544). Revealing the results of genetic tests can have implications for relatives as well as individuals. As sociologists have argued, genetic information challenges our ideas about personhood by emphasizing the connections and links between people, as it has implications both for the individual and for people to whom they are genetically related (Sommerville and English 1999).[3] However, in a liberal society the tendency is to locate control in the person from whom information is taken: 'to locate the control of this information solely with the sample source might, therefore, seem to many to be an inadequate response to concerns about how it should be treated' (Laurie 2002: 93).

While consent does not adequately reflect the interests of different family members in an individual's information, it is an essential requirement for research. The concept of autonomy that underpins consent is that of autonomous agents making their decisions on their own and according to their personal preferences. For Jennifer Nedelsky (1989) this is not a true account of autonomy, as it is never exercised in a vacuum: autonomy is a 'capacity that exists only in the context of social relations that support it and only in conjunction with the internal sense of being autonomous' (Nedelsky 1989: 7). Leslie Bender's study of decision-making in a medical context supports this view (Bender 1992). She argues that, in the medical context, to be autonomous and self-governing means that individuals' decisions are negotiated through a complex web of relationships of physicians and family members. Any information generated in this context is often formed in relationships with others, with all parties to that relationship having some claim to the information. Both these writers see autonomy as grounded not in isolation but in social relations with others. This has importance for genetics where information can have implications for more than just the individual. Therefore, if we value autonomy in genetic research, we must provide the circumstances to facilitate individual decision-making in consultation with other family members.

Despite the fact that consent does not adequately reflect the interests of different family members in an individual's information, it is very difficult to apply an alternative system that would recognize the familial interests in genetic information. The first problem with obtaining family consent is to define who is family, and second what would constitute family consent? In the case of Iceland where a genealogical database will be used in the population collection, the whole population could be established as related. Do we extend the notion of the family to all the people who can be traced to one ancestral couple or restrict it to only immediate family such as parents and siblings? In a population collection the immediate kin, such as parents, siblings and children, could be approached for permission to use an individual's DNA as a means of recognizing the familial nature of a sample. This would acknowledge that an individual is located within a series of relationships, all of which will have some implications on decision-making. However, not all families are united about the use of data and trying to seek consent from immediate kin is not always a straightforward process. This would also add to the administrative burden on the consent process. While the decision whether to be involved in a population collection currently rests with the individual, it should be understood that this decision should only be undertaken in consultation with other family members. Ways of recognizing this connection and allowing family members to be informed about the nature of the research and its implications should therefore be an important part of the procedures in a population collection.

Exceptions to informed consent

The difficulties of meeting the threshold requirements for consent and the inappropriateness of this for genetic research begs the question should we abandon the requirement for consent for population collections? In the medical context there are recognized exceptions to the requirement that informed consent must always be obtained. Some types of research, such as epidemiology that involves the study of traits across populations, have been conducted without informed consent because of the impracticalities of obtaining this consent (Last 1996). Genetic epidemiology and other research involving the study of large sample groups will be carried out on population collections. The justification for the lack of informed consent in epidemiology is often based on the principles of the public good, that there are benefits for society, and that there is minimal risk to the individual (Beauchamp 1996). It is regarded that if 'the research only involves minimal risk and will not adversely affect the rights and welfare of subjects beyond access to the data itself, then the research can occur without contacting subjects for actual consent' (Robertson 1998: 68). It is perceived that the risk to individuals is minimal because the research does not involve physical intervention and direct participation of the individual, but rather the use of information, which may often be statistical. This risk is further reduced through the removal of identifiers or rendering data anonymous. Therefore consequential arguments that emphasize the social good that will result from the research or the collection of information for public health purposes can often hold sway over rights-based arguments to protect the interests of individuals. Such infringements on autonomy have been accepted by society because of the benefits that will accrue to all by allowing the research to proceed (Foster 2001).

These principles are also found in European Union law in the public interest exemption under Directive 95/46/EC. The public interest exemption allows the processing of sensitive data in the public interest, for the purposes of 'preventive medicine, medical diagnosis, the provision of care or treatment or the management of health-care services' (Directive 95/46/EC Art. 8, para 3).[4] The research exemption under Directive 95/46/EC also allows information collected with consent to be further processed for new research projects without further consent of the individual and without providing information about the processing. This would solve the problem of trying to contact all the individuals in a population collection for every new research project. However, there are conditions attached to the exemption under Article 29 of the Directive 95/46/EC. Further research is only permitted if there are suitable safeguards in place that 'must in particular rule out the use of the data in support of measures or decisions regarding any particular individual' (Directive 95/46/EC Art. 29). This exemption allows research to be carried out on personal data without consent if the following conditions are fulfilled: that the disclosure of data for the purpose of a defined scientific research project concerning an important public interest has been authorized by the body or bodies designated by domestic law, but only if the data subject has not expressly opposed disclosure; despite reasonable efforts, it would be impracticable to contact the data subject to seek his consent; and the interests of the research project justify the authorization.

The public interest exemption allows the processing of identifiable data for a legitimate public purpose on the basis of 'opt-out'. While 'opt-out' was the standard of consent finally adopted by the *Althingi*, (the Icelandic Parliament) for the Icelandic population collection, there has been no legal challenge as to whether this conforms to human rights case law. To qualify for public interest exemption, research must come under areas specified in Directive 95/46/EC. Also, the measures for implementation must conform to the requirements of necessity and proportionality developed under the case law of the European Convention on Human Rights (1950). Therefore it is not clear whether opting out of a population collection would be regarded as an acceptable infringement on individual privacy on the basis of the public interest. There are also problems with applying the research exemption in the Directive 95/46/EC, as the research exemption only takes effect if information has already been collected with consent. As pointed out earlier, obtaining explicit and informed consent is not a straightforward process. Despite such difficulties, both these exemptions would allow information to be used without informed or explicit consent as long as this can be established to be in the public interest or for research purposes. So should these principles be applied to the collation of information in a population collection and secondary research on that information?

Applying these principles to population collections

If we suppose that exemptions to informed consent were to be applied to population collections, such a scenario could be justified on the following premises. Informed consent does not have to be sought for the collation of medical records, genealogies and DNA samples in population collections. These information sources are already accessed for a number of public interest purposes in the health service without consent. Therefore 'opt-out' is sufficient for the collation of information in a population collection that is largely derived from existing sources of information. The population collection would be established on the basis of 'opt-out' and informing individuals of the collection by putting up posters in hospitals and doctors' surgeries and using the media. As in epidemiological research the infringement of individual privacy is necessary, but would be minimal for the research to be carried out. The benefits of this research would be profound in helping researchers to understand the complex interplay between genes, as well as genes, environment and lifestyle that has implications for everyone in the population. The benefits of this research could revolutionize the way that treatment and diagnosis is carried out in the healthcare setting. Therefore the social benefits are high and the risks to individuals low – apart from the collection of one DNA sample (which would be obtained with consent and in future could be obtained from existing collections of biological samples), the use of genealogical information and existing information in medical records and health documents. For these reasons the public interest exemption should be applied to the collation of information in the population collection.

The safeguards in place would ensure that the risk of harm to individuals in using this information would be minimal. Medical professionals under an obligation of confidentiality would handle all data, and all patient contact would be through a healthcare worker. Individuals would have no active involvement in research as this would be conducted on previously collected information, and there would be no direct contact with researchers. A research ethics committee would give approval for secondary research use of the information. Once the data are collected personal identifiers would be removed and individuals will only be identifiable through an encrypted number, such as a National Health or National Identity number. This encryption would use the latest computer security safeguards to protect the data. This anonymization will mean that no harm would result to the participants in the population collection, and third parties would only be able to access statistical data from the population collection and so would not be able to receive information about specific individuals.

The size of the research sample makes it impractical and costly to seek the consent of all the people in the country, for the secondary use of information in the population collection. It may also be unethical to do so, in that it would worry people unnecessarily, or if consent were sought, people may not return the forms and the numbers would be too low to be statistically meaningful for population research purposes. As this research is not concerned with the individual but is about mapping trends within families and across the population, any secondary research should proceed without the informed or explicit consent of participants. I suggest that while these arguments are persuasive, it is with some reluctance that we should apply them to population collections.

Why these principles should not be applied to population collections

These principles have been accepted within medical research as the way to protect individual privacy, while allowing research in the public interest to be carried out. They represent a compromise of individual rights for the benefits that can accrue to all and should be used sparingly. Both privacy law and medical research practice recognize that if data is identifiable an individual has a strong moral claim to control its use, which needs strong public interest arguments to overturn. These exemptions therefore rest on a case for the public good being made, as well as a demonstration of minimal risk to individuals and that procedures are in place to anonymize data. Implicit within this exemption is the notion of the many checks and balances that are a part of the culture of medical research practice, which are a basis for the public trust essential to the functioning of medical research. In contrast to other population research it is not clear that population collections are in the public interest, or that risk to individuals is minimal and that data can be anonymized.

The primary aim of most commercial research is not to promote the health of society, but to develop research programmes that will bring in profits for shareholders and investors. The values that are implicit in a medical research culture located within a national health system do not have primacy in the context of a population collection. Whereas the medical research context is dependent upon trust and a belief that the research will have benefits for all, as well as a shared understanding of appropriate practice, this is not the case with population collections. The commercial nature of population collections highlights a dynamic that cannot be ignored. One of the main concerns about the Icelandic Health Sector Database is that the licence to operate the database will be in the hands of a private company, with the exclusive right to use it for financial gain. This means that the research agenda becomes susceptible to market changes and the need to attract investment rather than being free to address national health concerns. While it is anticipated that there will be long-term benefits to humanity as a whole by conducting research on population collections, many of the short-term benefits, such as intellectual property rights and profits will flow to the private company involved. It is difficult to argue that population collections are in the public interest when many of the benefits will not go to the population as a whole.

In a medical research context, giving up rights to control how information is further used in the public interest is more acceptable if information is given to specific researchers in relationships of trust with the individual. All the proposed population collections anticipate that access to the data will be given to third parties for a fee and that this will be a way of recovering many of the costs of establishing and maintaining the collection. Although data sharing does occur within the medical research context, the exclusive purpose is not to make money nor is it to allow access by multiple users. This has greater implications for privacy than does the sharing of data within a research team or between research teams where there are direct relationships between researchers and participants in the research project. This connection and the obligations that flow from and with it do not apply to data that are held within a population collection. Participants will have a different kind of relationship of trust with the doctor they have seen over many years than with a company that is not involved in their day-to-day healthcare management and is only interested in the data that are derived from this activity. Much of conventional medical research is conducted within a healthcare setting where the degree of trust is very high. The level of trust between an individual and a company that stands to gain a financial benefit out of the use of information is likely to be very different both in nature and degree. This adds a different flavour to the contextual integrity of population collections and distinguishes it from the medical research context that is based on a combination of ethical principles designed for the advancement of the public good within a healthcare setting.

The type of research carried out on a population collection will also be very different to conventional research practice. In a population collection data will continually be recycled and added to over time and the research uses will change as technology progresses. The information that is collected is not proportionate to the needs of one research project. In conventional research the research protocol must be specified and defined with a research hypothesis that will be tested in order to get ethics approval. Data are often kept by the researcher who has collected them and are only given to third parties for purposes such as public health, collaborative research or for auditing purposes. Information and samples will often be destroyed after the specific research project has finished or will be used by the same researcher but within the same restricted research area. In contrast, the main purposes of population collections are to be resource tools where data can be accumulated over time and can be accessed by a number of different users. The lawyer Henry Greely (2000) states that:

> The Health Sector Database law, and deCODE's plans, would not ask a person to participate in a particular research protocol, but instead to become part of a resource, used for many protocols, concerning many different protocols, concerning many different medical conditions.
>
> (Greely 2000: 179, n. 93)

The purpose of a population collection is to 'mine' the data for associations and then to follow up with specific research projects. The nature of future research will change as technology increases and as there are further advances in genomic research.

Population collections, as opposed to other types of population research, present greater risks to research participants in terms of risk of harm. The possibility of harm is heightened by the fact that genetic information will be used and linked to other sources of personal information. The process of a researcher searching through medical records is very different from the risk of harm when genetic information and other personal information is combined to create a comprehensive profile on individuals, families and other groups in society. The aggregation of a number of different information sources means that a profile of an individual can be gleaned from this process that may be very different from that obtained from using only one data source. The addition of genealogies in a population collection means that family profiles may be discerned as well as individual profiles. Information that seems perfectly innocuous in one context takes on a new dimension when it is collated, because together this information provides a different picture, or perspective of an individual and their family. While this offers enormous research potential, 'the information in these linked databases would be more sensitive than the isolated bits of information contained in particular disease registries' (Greely 2000: 180). The effect of collating data is to make data that are non-sensitive in one context – such as hospital admission dates – highly sensitive when they are linked to genetic information or medical records. This allows a comprehensive picture of someone's potential and current personal medical information to be compiled. Therefore the collation of data increases the sensitivity of all information in the population collection and the potential risk to individuals as the collation gives the data a new value and potency.

There will never be minimal risk to individuals whose information is in a population collection as the data will always be identifiable and this will increase over time as more data accumulate. This is because there must be some way of identifying the individual in order to link data and because of their quality and comprehensiveness. The encrypting of individual identifiers cannot be used to render information in a population collection anonymous and therefore minimize risk. Therefore the individual's moral right to control the use of personal information increases over time, and as more sources of information are collated. This imposes a moral obligation on the receiver of the data to treat them with respect, and to inform the individual as to how information will be used, but also distinguishes population collections from other research projects. Moreover, as DNA is a unique identifier, this makes it very difficult to anonymize data in a population collection (Green and Thomas 1998). Individuals have a unique genome sequence that distinguishes them from the rest of humanity and can be derived from a DNA sample.[5] As Thomas Murray (1997) states, 'although the practice of removing identifying information is usually thought to confer anonymity by making the records impossible to trace to an individual, that may not be the case with records containing significant chunks of sequence data' (Murray 1997). The population geneticist Bryan Sykes (Sykes and Irven 2000) argues that he can identify male individuals in his family by matching DNA patterns on their Y chromosome (Gray 2002). If this can be achieved through the analysis of DNA then the removal of an individual's name as a means of safeguarding privacy is potentially redundant. Therefore the most common means of protecting privacy by removing personal identifiers may be effectual in the short term, but may have limited effectiveness when there are sequences of whole genomes to compare. This means that there needs to be careful consideration of the safeguards needed to protect privacy and to ensure that these are continually developed to keep up with technological changes. In medical research the encryption of data has been used as a basis for minimizing risk; while this can be used in population collections it cannot be the only form of protection as the data are also indirectly identifiable.

The fact that population collections contain DNA samples and genetic information in the form of computerized sequence codes, family histories and genealogies increases the potential risks to participants. While a medical diagnosis may be specific to the individual, a genetic diagnosis may also indicate risks for other family members (Gostin 1998). Therefore the analysis of one person's DNA could point to factors relevant to another family member's health.

Genetic information is also regarded as sensitive information because of the potential to use it as a basis for discrimination in areas such as employment and insurance (Annas 1993, Murray 1997, Holm 1999). In Iceland, there has been much debate as to whether insurance companies would be able to use the Health Sector Database and if they were, what type of questions they would be allowed to ask. Therefore genetic information has been perceived as creating higher risks for individuals because it can confirm certain diseases for individuals, as well as family members, but also it has the potential to be used as a basis for discrimination in insurance and employment.

The use of DNA samples in population collection also increases the possibility of risk for individuals, because it is impossible to foresee all the potential uses of DNA. One DNA sample could yield a whole genome sequence for an individual, as well as 'information to study any and all genes, as well as the information to do a genetic fingerprint' (Murray 1997: 64). Therefore the information contained within one DNA sample can be used for a number of different research applications just because of the comprehensiveness of the information contained within the sample. It is possible to splice an individual DNA sequence and use various parts of it, such as genes that have specific functions, to ask unrelated research questions from the same sample. So one sample can be used for many research applications, many of which are not necessarily anticipated at the present time. It is argued that developments in technology and research will enable us to apply to understand the implications of this information with greater accuracy and precision (Juengst 1991, Rachinsky 2000). As Pall Hriennson states:

> Given the rate at which technology is forging ahead in this field, we can be sure that in another ten years it will be possible to read far more from DNA samples than we can read today [. . .] DNA samples are like a mine that we are just beginning to work, and as yet we have only a very limited idea of the riches that may be recovered from it later on.
>
> (Hreinnson 2000: 4)

If properly stored there is no limit to the longevity of biological samples and the possible tests carried out on them in the future. The limitation is simply on the amount of sample that is available for experimentation: 'in some cases, these preserved remains from past or current genetic studies may outlive the individuals who donated them' (Green and Thomas 1998: 57). It is also possible because of the living nature of DNA that cell lines can be grown from them, which could be replicated and used indefinitely for research such as the Mo or HeLa cell lines (Landecker 1999a, 1999b). There can be multiple secondary use of samples without the knowledge and consent of tissue sources. Using current techniques the best DNA samples are derived from blood samples. Most of the proposed population collections will use genetic information that has been derived from individual samples of 50 millilitres of blood. To obtain DNA material for genetic testing there does not need to be the invasion of the body, a private space, or a relationship (Lombardo 1996). As Martin Richards notes, 'this makes it easy to carry out DNA tests without the knowledge and consent of the person involved' (Richards 2001: 682). Therefore a population collection holding DNA samples on a population will be able to use such samples for many kinds of research projects that will increase with further development of appropriate techniques.

The combination of all of these factors has privacy implications for the person who is donating a DNA sample. If an individual is consenting to the use of a medical record, he or she will have been involved in, or aware of most of the activities and observations that have been recorded. Therefore an individual will have a fair idea of the implications of the use of the information contained within the medical record. In contrast, it is impossible to know the extent of the information that is held within a DNA sample and its implications for the individual. I would argue that in the case of a medical record, the individual will have a far better understanding of what they are consenting to, than when they consent to the use of a DNA sample. This suggests that protections applying to the use of DNA samples should be greater than those to the use of medical records and should be updated as research technology advances. However the present situation is that:

> The regulations on the processing of personal data are far clearer than those applying to the acquisition and preservation of biosamples. If we are to ensure the legal protection of genetic privacy, we must guarantee that clear and well grounded regulations apply to the acquisition and preservation of biosamples, and also to the processing of data from those samples.
>
> (Hriennson 2000: 2)

The concern is that if such information is collated without the full knowledge and consent of the people involved, this may have the effect of forcing people to limit their behaviour and thereby restrict their freedom. In Iceland there were concerns that patients would no longer be able to give information to a physician for treatment and diagnosis without that being recorded on the population collection's database (Berger 1999). This process moves sensitive information out of the intimate realms of the physician/patient relationship into that of a public record, which can be accessed by people that are unknown to the individual. Therefore, giving information to a doctor becomes a different and more complex activity. This use of personal data could force individuals to act differently with their doctor, and to exclude details important to medical care on the basis that this may be passed on to third parties. This means that not only are the acts of individuals changed because they may be concerned about access to that information, but also their freedom is limited. Therefore the state is under an obligation to ensure that population collections are not used for unauthorized purposes, by informing the population of the kind of information that will be collected and restricting the purposes for which it will be used.

What principles should we have for population collections?

Arguably, population collections present greater risks to individuals than have been posed by other kinds of population research carried out in the public interest within the medical context. Therefore I contend that it is not possible to apply the public exemption or the research exemption to population collections because they do not pose minimal risk. This means that consent should be obtained and the individual has a moral right to control how such information is used. However, as discussed earlier, it is difficult to obtain explicit or informed consent for the collation of information in a population collection and for every new research use of the population collection. The fact that moral obligation to the individual will increase over time as profiles are built and the data becomes more identifiable means that some kind of consent is necessary for the use of this data. While it is only possible to obtain broad consent when the information is first collated for entry onto the population collection, this broad consent cannot also apply to all other research conducted on the population collection. Once the researchers and the type of research is known there is a moral obligation to give this information to individuals and to allow them to make a decision as to whether their information should be used for such purposes. The nature of genetic information means there is an obligation to accommodate the interests of the family as well as the other groups in society and that of the population as a whole. So what rights does this give to people whose information is on a population collection?

When information is first collected, individuals would be required to consent to the use of information in the population collection and the fact that this will be linked to other databases. They should be informed of the organization in charge of data collection, the types of data that would be processed, as well as a broad description of the researchers and the type of research planned. While this cannot be specific enough to conform to the requirements of explicit consent, it is as close as the circumstances will allow. Every new type of information collected from the individual or other sources for entry into the population collection must be accompanied with consent. The complex and sensitive nature of the data, as well as the fact that they will increase over time in quality and sensitivity, means that individuals should have a right to know what information is held about them. The individual would have the right to stop information going onto the population collection as well as having the right to withdraw from the population collection at any time. If this was exercised, all information on the individual would have to be deleted from the different databases and any DNA samples would have to be destroyed. Every individual would have to re-consent to the use of the data in the population collection every five years. This would be a re-consent to the continued use of existing data and the use of the new accumulated personal data in the population collection. It would also impose an obligation on the controllers of the population collection to explain any changes in use or research strategy of the project.

To make sure individuals were able to exercise their choice over the information in the population collection there would need to be a sufficient range of options for people to choose from. One way to do this would be to send all participants regular information on the research planned on the population collection, in the form of a newsletter for example, which could also be available on the Internet and through health centres. This would ensure that individuals are kept informed about the future research uses of the data, when the details of the research are known. On the basis of this individuals could choose whether they would become involved in specific research projects. The exercise of choice cannot be on the basis of a positive consent because of the sheer impracticalities of applying this. Therefore consent for secondary use would be on the basis of opting out of projects rather than opting in. If individuals fail to 'opt-out' of a research project within the required time, then information would be included in a study. This option would allow individuals to regulate how their information can be used, with reasonable certainty that this will be retained in the future. 'Opt-out' for the secondary use of information is acceptable as long as individuals can obtain information about the research and there are systems of data protection, such as oversight committees and restricted access to data on the population collection.

While 'opt-out' is a practical solution to the issue of consent it does not allow control over the information in the population collection at a level that would be usually required for the degree of sensitivity of the information held in the population collection. This is a compromise between protecting individual privacy and allowing information to be used for the public good. Given the sensitivity of the data, additional safeguards must be in place to protect individual privacy. While consent addresses the issue of respecting the individual, it does not acknowledge that information in the population collection also has implications for people other than the individual. Consent is an individual concern and it is impossible to give voice to the concerns of other family members, a group or those of a nation. It is also limited in its scope, as while it allows people to say yes or no to research projects, it does not determine which research makes it onto the agenda. The problem of the consent model is that it does not bring into question the legitimacy of the initial request itself. Therefore, there must be other mechanisms in place in order to deal with the wider issues of information gathering at the population level as well as ensuring that the priorities of the population collection are those of the community.

Beyond informed consent: additional safeguards for population collections

One of the issues with population research is how to make participants aware of the issues that may affect them as a group rather than just as individuals. Responding to the political difficulties encountered by the Human Genome Diversity Project in the 1990s, an ethics body commissioned by its organizers suggested that 'both the group and individuals should be consulted before the undertaking of research' (North American Regional Committee, Human Genome Diversity Project 1997). It is important for the population as a whole to assess the social implications of establishing such a comprehensive body of sensitive information, and to decide upon issues such as access by third parties and whether uses other than medical research should be allowed. Thorough community consultation should also engage the population 'as partners in planning and carrying out the research and not just as research subjects' (North American Regional Committee, Human Genome Diversity Project 1997). Community consultation enables people to debate these issues in a meaningful and inclusive way, before a collection is established, 'either through the democratic process or through the media' (Knoppers 2001: 3). This approach would treat the population as participants in the research, and would acknowledge their contribution. It would also allow the public to be involved in planning the population collection and in deciding whether it should be allowed to proceed. Patient groups could help to set the agenda of research that would mean that individuals would have had the opportunity to frame the research questions that they would be consenting to. Being able to understand research in a wider perspective enables individuals to be more informed about research, before deciding whether to give individual consent. This helps to compensate for the inability to obtain informed or explicit consent for the establishment and subsequent research on the population collection. But how should these principles be put into practice?

For an 'opt-out' system to be legitimate there must be other ways of recognizing the interests of the people who have information on the population collection. A suggestion has been made that one alternative to consent may be the use of representatives (Baumrind 1978). These representatives would be on the committees that approve research projects and oversee the running of the population collection. This would give a perspective in the decision-making process that represents that of the people whose information is used in the population collection. So rather than individuals being asked to consent to particular options, in this model they would be instrumental in formulating the options and would be involved in determining which research would be conducted. Such representatives would provide the litmus test for understanding when the 'people in the subject population take the view that certain aspects of their lives are particularly private matters, onto which the researchers should be especially reluctant to intrude' (Capron 1991: 86S). They would also be able to be involved in determining the long-term strategy for the population collection. Therefore the people who had information in the population collection could influence the type of research questions asked as well as the running of the management structures.

One of the concerns with population collections is that the involvement of private companies and market forces may mean that these can be sold as part of a company's assets. If we are serious about respecting privacy then opportunities for control over information must be in the hands of the people from whom it was obtained. If data are accumulating over decades, many of the donors of information will die or cease to have the capacity to consent in a meaningful way. There needs to be a structure that can protect the interests of these people, as well as the population as a whole, which can span generations and exist in perpetuity. One such legal mechanism is that of a trust, which could hold the legal title to information and be run by trustees. All information would be placed in a trust for perpetuity and the trustees overseeing the information would act on behalf of the people who had altruistically provided information to the population collection. They would be accountable to individuals but could also act as representatives for the community as a whole.

The benefits of a trust are that it would acknowledge the fact that genetic information has a number of dimensions to it. Genetic information at the collective level, the human genome shared by us all, has been posited to be 'the common heritage of humanity' (UNESCO Declaration, 1997 Art. 1). I argue that this is an interest that should be properly respected and protected. At the same time, at the personal level, it is unique, belonging to the individual, as well as being information that has implications for other family members. Therefore it is important that such information is properly cared for and can be protected for future generations. Placing the control of information in the hands of the trustees who have a legal obligation to individuals also means that information will stay within the community. Such mechanisms should protect against harm and ensure the security of data so that people will have confidence in entrusting information to a population collection. A trust keeps this information as a resource for the country rather than being bought and sold subject to market forces. It also means that ownership is retained by the individuals who have donated information, which would at the same time respect and acknowledge their contribution.

There is a tendency to focus on consent as the means to protect privacy, which ignores the fact that there also need to be technical, procedural and supervisory mechanisms to maintain security of data and public confidence in population collections. If an individual is giving intimate data for medical research, they need to be certain of the trustworthiness of the institution to which they give information. Mechanisms need to be in place to ensure security of data through encryption and security measures, and supervisory bodies with appropriate powers of enforcement to ensure that these procedures are followed. There needs to be separately constituted bodies to oversee the establishment and running of the database, with clear separation of duties and responsibilities and powers of enforcement and supervision. Such a structure ensures that the handling of the raw data, the encryption of data, and enforcement and management of the population collection are carried out by different organizations. This transparency, combined with very tight technical computer procedures and requirements, builds public confidence in the population collection. The managers of the population collection need to 'offer individuals simple and realistic ways of checking what they consent to is indeed what happens, and what they do not consent to does not happen' (O'Neill 2001: 702). Such procedures ensure that privacy can be maintained and while they are not a substitute for allowing individual's choice about their private matters, they make it possible for information to be used in the public interest without infringing privacy.

Conclusion

The principles that have been developed in the medical context for population research cannot be readily applied to population collections and population genetics research. This is because the research strategy, the researchers and the research motives of population collections are very different to conventional research. Population collections do not represent minimal risk to participants because they will contain genetic information and will develop profiles on individuals and families over time. The information in the population collection will always be identifiable, and will increase over time as more data are accumulated. This has privacy implications for individuals as well as other family members and different groups in society.

In the world of genomics, advances in technology can mean rapid change in the information that can be derived from a DNA sample and what it can tell us about disease susceptibility. This research can have implications for individuals in terms of insurance, employment and family relations. Therefore it is not possible to hand a DNA sample or access to personal information over to researchers in perpetuity, without allowing the individual some control over what happens to the sample or the accumulated personal information in the future. The public interest and research exemption would effectively allow this to happen on the basis of 'opt-out'. The Icelandic population collection was established on this basis and was condemned by the international community and vocal opponents within Iceland.

This chapter has presented an alternative way to recognize individual as well as family and community rights over information in a population collection that is not based on explicit and informed consent and the exemptions that have been allowed in the public interest for research. These mechanisms are more appropriate for the new context of population collections and the use of collated information for secondary genetic research as they recognize the interests in the information in a population collection and that these interests will continue over time.

Notes

1. Population collections provide an administrative structure for the collection, collation, storage, linking and use of different types of personal information in collections, derived from a combination of primary sources such as medical records, questionnaires, DNA samples and genealogies. The aim is to add information to a collection over time as individuals seek healthcare treatment, as children are born and people die. This means that the quality and complexity of the information held on both the individual and the population as a whole will increase over time. Information within the population collection can be kept for many years and used for multiple, secondary research purposes by different researchers at the same time.
2. Directive 95/46/EC has been implemented in the UK by the Data Protection

Act 1998 and in other European states by their respective data protection legislation.

3. For a sociological discussion of the potential impact of genetic knowledge on discourses of personhood, especially in the context of genetic testing, see Hallowell (1999) and Kenen (1994).

4. The conditions that are attached to this exemption are that: it must be a defined scientific research project concerning an important public interest; data must be processed by a health professional subject to the rules of confidentiality or someone with an equivalent obligation; there must be suitable safeguards in place; data subjects should be entitled to object to the processing of any data relating to her/himself (Directive 95/46/EC Recital 45); and that any exemptions must be specified 'either by national law or by decision of the supervisory authority' and should be notified to the European Commission (Directive 95/46/EC Art. 8, para 6).

5. The exceptions to this are monozygotic twins who do share identical genome sequences.

References

Annas, G.J. (1993). 'Privacy rules for DNA databanks – protecting coded "Future Diaries"', *Journal of the American Medical Association* 270: 2346–2350.

Baumrind, D. (1978). 'Nature and definition of informed consent in research involving deception', in National Commission for the Protection of Human Subjects of Biomedical and Behavioral Research. *The Belmont Report: Ethical Principles and Guidelines for the Protection of Human Subjects of Research*, DHEW Publication No. (OS) 78–0014. Washington, D.C.: Government Printing Office; Appendix, Vol. 2, pp. 23–42.

Beauchamp, T.L. (1996). 'Moral foundations', in S. Coughlin and T.L. Beauchamp (eds) *Ethics and Epidemiology*, Oxford: Oxford University Press.

Bender, L. (1992). 'A feminist analysis of physician-assisted dying and voluntary active euthanasia', *Tennessee Law Review* 59: 519–547.

Berger, A. (1999). 'Private company wins rights to Icelandic gene database', *British Medical Journal* 318: 11.

Capron, A.M. (1991). 'Protection of research subjects: do special rules apply in epidemiology?' *Journal of Clinical Epidemiology* 44(Suppl. 1): 81S–89S.

Directive 95/46/EC on the Protection of Individuals with Regard to Automatic Processing of Personal Data. Online. Available HTTP: <http://www.dataprivacy.ie/6aii.htm>.

Dolgin, J.L. (2000). 'Choice, tradition and the new genetics: the fragmentation of the ideology of family', *Connecticut Law Review* 32: 523–566.

Foster, C. (2001) *The Ethics of Medical Research on Human Beings*, Cambridge: Cambridge University Press.

Gostin, L.O. (1995). 'Health information privacy', *Cornell Law Review* 80: 451–528.

Gray, C. (2002). '10 numbers that can trace your family tree', *The Independent*, 10 August 2002, London.

Greely, H.T. (2000). 'Iceland's plans for genomic research: facts and implications', *Jurimetrics* 40: 153–191.

Green, R.M. and Thomas, M.A. (1998). 'DNA: five distinguishing features for policy analysis', *Harvard Journal of Law and Technology* vol. 11(3), Summer 1998: 571.

Hallowell, N. (1999). 'Doing the right thing: genetic risk and responsibility', in P. Conrad and J. Gabe (eds) *Sociological Perspectives on the New Genetics*, Oxford: Blackwell.

Holm, S. (1999). 'There is nothing special about genetic information', in A.K. Thompson and R.F. Chadwick (eds) *Genetic Information Acquisition, Access and Control*, New York: Kluwer Academic/Plenum Publishers.

Hreinnson, P. (2000). 'The protection of genetic privacy', paper presented at 22nd International Conference on Privacy and Data Protection, Venice.

Human Genome Organisation (HUGO) Ethics Committee (2000). Statement on benefit-sharing. London: Human Genome Organisation.

Juengst, E.T. (1991). 'Priorities in professional ethics and social policy for human genetics', *Journal of the American Medical Association* 266: 1835–1836.

Kenen, R. (1994). 'The Human Genome Project: creator of the potentially sick, potentially vulnerable and potentially stigmatized?' in I. Robinson (ed.) *Life and Death under High Technology Medicine*, Colloquium. London: Manchester University Press and Fulbright Commission.

Knoppers, B.M. (2001). 'Of population, genetics and banks', *Genetics Law Monitor* Jan/Feb: 3–6.

Landecker, H. (1999a). 'Between beneficence and chattel: the human biological in law and science', *Science in Context* 12: 203–225.

Landecker, H. (1999b). 'Immortality, *in vivo*: a history of the HeLa cell line', in P. Brodwin (ed.) *Biotechnology, Culture, and the Body*, Bloomington: Indiana UP.

Last, J. (1996) 'Professional standards of conduct for epidemiologists' in S. Covelin and T.L. Beauchamp (eds) *Ethics and Epidemiology*, Oxford: Oxford University Press.

Laurie, G.T. (2002). *Genetic Privacy a Challenge to Medico-Legal Norms*, Cambridge: Cambridge University Press.

Lombardo, P.A. (1996). 'Genetic confidentiality: what's the big secret', *University of Chicago Law School Roundtable* 3: 589–615.

Murray, T.H. (1997). 'Genetic exceptionalism and "future diaries": Is genetic information different from other medical information?' in M.A. Rothstein (ed.) *Genetic Secrets: Protecting Privacy and Confidentiality in the Genetic Era*, New Haven: Yale University Press.

Nedelsky, J. (1989). 'Reconceiving autonomy: sources, thoughts and possibilities', *Yale Journal of Law and Feminism* 1: 7–14.

North American Regional Committee of the Human Genome Diversity Project (1997). 'Model protocol proposed ethical protocol for collecting DNA samples', *Houston Law Review* 33: 1431–1473.

O'Neill, O. (2001). 'Informed consent and genetic information', *Studies in the History and Philosophy of Biological and Biomedical Sciences* 32: 689–704.

Rachinsky, T.L. (2000). 'Genetic testing: toward a comprehensive policy to prevent genetic discrimination in the workplace', *University of Pennsylvania Journal of Labor and Employment Law* 2: 575–631.

Richards, M. (2001). 'How distinctive is genetic information?' *Studies in History and Philosophy of Biological and Biomedical Sciences* 32: 663–687.

Robertson, J.A. (1999). 'Privacy issues in second stage genomics', *Jurimetrics* 40(Fall): 59–75.

Sommerville, A. and English, V. (1999). 'Genetic privacy: orthodoxy or oxymoron?' *Journal of Medical Ethics* 25: 144–150.

Sykes, B. and Irven, C. (2000). 'Surnames and the Y chromosome', *The American Journal of Human Genetics* 66: 1417–1419.

UNESCO Universal Declaration on the Human Genome and Human Rights (1997). Available: http://www.unesco.org/ibc/en/genome/projet/index.htm.

World Medical Association (2000). Declaration of Helsinki Ethical Principles for Medical Research Involving Human Subjects, 52nd WMA General Assembly, Edinburgh, Scotland, October 2000. Available: http://www.wma.net/e/policy/b3.htm.

Chapter 8

Children's participation in genetic epidemiology

Consent and control

Emma Williamson, Trudy Goodenough, Julie Kent and Richard Ashcroft

Introduction

This chapter is about how child and parent participants in the Avon Longitudinal Study of Parents and Children (ALSPAC), a longitudinal genetic epidemiological study operating in the UK, view ethical protection. During the course of the research that we have undertaken, we spoke with both children and parents about the long term use of data 'given' for research purposes. This chapter will analyse the views of both groups and identify where differences arose. First, we will examine how children perceive the decision-making process and the amount of control they have within it in comparison with the views of parents. Second, we consider the legal and ethical 'rights' of parents to consent to the long term use of their children's biological and genetic information for research. And finally, we discuss how child participants perceive notions of 'risk' with regard to different types of information and how this might influence the validity of the proxy consent process. The overall objective in doing our research was to discuss ethical issues relating to health research with the participating children in a meaningful way. We were clear from the outset that we wished to talk with the children in a way that did not impose adult-centred approaches to knowledge and understanding. Society is changing, children across the world are increasingly viewed, theoretically at least, as active participants in society and accorded 'rights' (United Nations 1989). By seeking to illustrate the perceptions of children on issues that affect them, this chapter raises concerns about the limitations of proxy consent in relation to the long term use of biological and genetic information. However, it is not specifically concerned with the issue of competence. Competence is discussed, where relevant, in relation to the legal criteria for competency, but we are not discussing here whether children are competent to make these decisions on their own or not. We discuss shared decision-making, and outline how the views of children can inform the way in which they are asked to participate in research.

The ALSPAC study

ALSPAC, also known as the 'Children of the 90s' study, is an extensive epidemiological genetic longitudinal study of children born in the Avon area with an expected date of delivery between 1 April 1991 and 31 December 1992. The specific aim of ALSPAC is:

> To determine ways in which biological, environmental, social, psycho-logical and psychosocial factors are associated with the survival and optimal health and development of the foetus, infant and child, and ways in which the causal relationships might vary with the genetic composition of the mother and/or child. ALSPAC has the long-term aim of following the children into adulthood to answer questions related to prenatal and postnatal factors associated, for example with schizophrenia, delinquency, reproductive failure on the one hand and realization of full educational potential, health and happiness on the other.
>
> (ALSPAC 2002)

ALSPAC began as part of the World Health Organization's European Longitudinal Study of Pregnancy and Childhood (ELSPAC).

> In the early 1980s, the WHO Regional Office for Europe included in its programme of support, the epidemiological investigation of factors influencing child health and development. The main reason for this was that there was insufficient knowledge available to develop effective disease prevention strategies in early life, particularly in relation to behavioural, environmental and social factors.
>
> (ELSPAC 2003a)

There are currently seven countries participating in the ELSPAC study, the Czech Republic, Greece, the Isle of Man, Russia, Slovakia, the Ukraine and the UK. Comparisons of recruitment rates across the different regions are difficult due to: different healthcare provision, and thus opportunity to recruit all pregnant women; emigration; divorce rates, which make contact with biological fathers difficult; and finally, in some regions, a lack of interest (ELSPAC 2003b).

Within the ALSPAC study in the UK, 14,893 pregnancies[1] were enrolled in the study of which 13,955 are still being followed, accounting for 14,138 children. The actual enrolment rate among eligible mothers is thought to be between 80 and 90 per cent (ELSPAC 2003b). ALSPAC collects information from parents and children in a number of ways; self-completion questionnaires; hands-on assessment in a standardized environment;[2] medical, educational and other records; biological samples from the mother, partner and child; and in-depth interviews and observations of particular subgroups and their controls

(Golding *et al.* 2001). It also offers additional involvement to the children via 'the Discovery Club'[3] and children's web pages, and to parents with Newsletters and the parent website. The ALSPAC study has been funded from a variety of sources since it started. These include the University of Bristol where the ALSPAC study is located, the Wellcome Trust, the Medical Research Council, the Department of Health, the Department of the Environment as well as other government bodies, charitable research organizations, commercial companies and individual sponsorship.[4]

Since its inception ALSPAC has collected a range of biological samples from both children and parents. These include: maternal blood, maternal urine, cord blood, umbilical cord, placentas, hair and nail clippings, teeth, child's blood, DNA and urine. Child's blood, if both parents and children agree, was taken at 7 years of age and it is planned to take (with permission) further blood samples at ages 9, 11, 13, and 15 years of age from the children (ALSPAC 2003b). In addition,

> DNA will be aliquoted for all mothers and children for whom permission is received. The DNA is obtained for the mother from maternal blood samples already collected, and for the child from the umbilical cord, from cord blood and from further blood samples or buccal samples taken later in childhood. Funding has now been obtained to take blood from those parents and children who are willing to have their cell lines transformed and thus allow an unlimited source of DNA.
>
> (ALSPAC 2003a)

The biological samples which ALSPAC has collected serve a number of purposes:

> Biological samples are of great importance to the study for a variety of different reasons: (a) they can be a source of DNA; (b) they provide information about mechanisms linking genetic variation to phenotypes; (c) they can provide phenotypes in themselves and (d) they provide biomarkers for exposure to a variety of pollutants (e.g. pesticides, trace metals).
>
> (ALSPAC 2003b)

In relation to the collection of personal data and information, in addition to the measurements taken when parents and children visit the study, parents began completing questionnaires prior to the child's birth and have continued to do so over the past 11 years. As such there is a vast amount of personal information held by the ALSPAC study which has enabled the study to examine nutrition, asthma, allergies and atopic disorders, obesity and growth, mental health of parents, child development, temperament and behaviour, physical environment, vision and hearing. In addition to the ALSPAC study's primary objectives, a number of sub-studies, involving subpopulations of the ALSPAC cohort have examined: child language delay, air pollution, alcohol and breast-feeding, day care, peanut allergies, family type and the impact of having brothers and sisters.

As this brief description of the ALSPAC study shows, this is a vast study which has incorporated the collection of both biological, genetic, and non-biological, non-genetic information about the study families over the course of the last 11 years. It is from this cohort that participants in our research were recruited. Although this research focuses on participants of the ALSPAC study, the arguments in this paper relate to the ethical dilemmas that arise in the collection of material for research databases generally and not specifically to the ALSPAC study itself.

The EPEG project

The research discussed in this chapter was carried out as part of the EPEG Project (Ethical Protection in Epidemiological Genetic Research: Participants' Perspectives), which started in October 2000 and is due for completion in October 2003. Funded by the Wellcome Trust, the aim of the EPEG project is to improve understanding of the ethical issues in epidemiological research, with special reference to clinical genetics, to longitudinal studies, and to research involving children. The project team brings together researchers and theorists from a number of disciplinary backgrounds including: medical and bioethics, sociology, psychology, social policy and child development. In addition to the project team, the project's advisory group adds to the multidisciplinary approach by bringing to the project philosophers, medics, epidemiologists, lawyers and lay representatives. In relation to this chapter we sought to improve our understanding of children's capacity to make decisions about their own participation in genetic and other clinical testing in non-therapeutic research, and explore the factors influencing initial and continued participation by adults and children in longitudinal studies.

Participants in the EPEG project were recruited from four distinct groups: children aged 8–11 years old who have participated in the ALSPAC study since prior to their birth; mothers, who were primary carers of children enrolled in the study; fathers, who were partners to study mothers; and parents of children of a same age cohort who do not take part in the ALSPAC study.

The EPEG project consisted of two distinct phases: the first phase included focus groups with the four sample groups; the second one-to-one interviews. Between October 2000 and 2002 nine focus groups were facilitated ($n = 35$) and 132 one-to-one interviews were conducted.

The methodological tools used within each phase and with adult and child participants included innovative as well as traditional focus group and interview methodologies (Williamson *et al.* 2001). We were clear from the outset that we did not wish to 'test' the children and attempted throughout to enable the children, rather than us as adults/researchers, to define the issues that they considered important and relevant to their experiences of research participation (Goodenough *et al.* 2003). Both adults and children were asked a range of questions about research, confidentiality, consent, participation, and about different types of information or data. With regard to the long term use of data and information, adult participants were specifically asked about consent for use, whether they felt the need for further 'protective' measures within longitudinal research, and whether they felt that the collection and use of different types of information (genetic/non-genetic) made a difference. Parents and children were also asked about issues related to consent and proxy consent or decision-making.

Most of the children did not raise, or appear to be specifically interested in, the area of genetics. As such, in keeping with our methodological approach, children were asked wider questions about the types of information they give to the ALSPAC study, the way it is collected and kept, and how they would feel about the information being used by a similar project in the future. This enabled us to explore the views of children about the long term use of their information.

The act and process of participation

Prior to addressing specific research findings it is important to understand how children and adults perceive their research participation in relation to the long term use of genetic and non-genetic information. When asked about how the data they had 'given' to research might be used both now and in the future, children related it to both personal and wider benefits.

Participant: They might either keep it and test and keep testing it with other people like do 'Children of 2000' and stuff like that or they might burn it.

(Male child aged 9)

This example is interesting as it describes comparing the data which ALSPAC children have given with that derived from a later hypothetical study which matches the study they have been participating within. The alternative proposition that the study might 'burn it' (their information), relates to this child's view of how confidentiality will be achieved by destroying the data.

Participant: I think that they're going to, well actually I'm really strange you see, because I've got big imaginations so like I think like they're going to pass them into the future so I'm going to be known forever and ever so is other people.
Interviewer: Who are they going to pass them to into the future?
Participant: Like other scientists, other people like, I'm assume then it's nearly

completely finished, I'm like really old like they're going to pass them to scientists and they're going to just keep them on one big record and then some day they're just going to say about 'these are the Children of the 90s' and they're going to pass them down to the school so they have to learn about Children of the 90s.

Interviewer: Sounds a bit like a history.

Participant: Yeah the history.

(Female child aged 10)

This extract locates the future use of data within a wider notion of both science and history. This child believes they will be 'known forever' and that children in the future will have to learn about her and the other 'Children of the 90s' at school.

Participant: Well I think they're keeping it in storage, if I come, they'll know about me, they'll know what I like, know what I don't like.

Interviewer: And what do you think about them hanging on to it like that?

Participant: Um, I think its good like that because there's less things they get wrong and more things they get right.

(Male child aged 9)

This extract highlights an issue talked about by a number of children, which raises questions about the ways in which children understand the concept of anonymity. This child believes that by keeping data the study will use the information to tailor future study focus sessions (where children visit the study for a range of tests to be carried out) to their likes and dislikes. Other children who talked about the use of data in a similar way described their perception of the data and information being kept in large folders with the child's name on it. In some cases they believed that this folder would be returned to them at a later date and expressed the view that this would be very interesting to them.

Interviewer: Okay, so what do you think will happen to all your information in the future? Say the study stopped when you were fifteen or sixteen but they still had all your information, what do you think they would do with it?

Participant: I think they'd probably keep it 'cause like things like police profiles.

(Male child aged 10)

This participant suggests that the data could be put to other purposes such as police profiling. Again this raises questions about whether some of the children are informed about or understand the boundaries of the research, anonymity and accessibility of their data.

Parents were asked about the use of genetic information in research, forensic and medical databases. In the majority of interviews adult participants considered the merits of each potential use and did not consider it appropriate for data collected for one purpose to be used in another without their consent being sought.

> I don't trust the [genetic] profiling and because that is data that is, once it's out there, it's impossible to recall. Lifestyle stuff can change, characters do change, rarely, less so as you get on in life, but nonetheless people can be faced with life threatening situations that causes a complete re-evaluation of where they are. So lifestyle things change, your genetic information won't change, unless we start talking about stem cells. But yet that information won't change so if that information is out there about you, that is it, and how do you recall it? You can't.
>
> (ALSPAC father)

> *Interviewer*: Is there anything else that you've chosen not to take part in?
> *Participant*: Yeah the cell line, I chose not to do . . . I think I was happy for him to give, it doesn't actually bother him giving blood . . . because at some stage in your life you're going to have to do some kind of medical test probably . . . But I felt uncomfortable with the cell lines because I felt that's something, I'm giving permission for something, some part of my son that would go on for years and years and years, and I didn't feel confident about giving permission for that. If it was about me, then that would be my decision, but I was making that decision for him, and it would go on until, that would go on forever, those cell lines, until he was old enough to make his own decision, and I didn't feel comfortable about doing that.
>
> (ALSPAC mother)

Both of these extracts illustrate some of the fears and concerns which parents expressed when discussing the long term use of genetic information in research. Time plays an important factor in their own consent and decision-making processes and, as a consequence, in their proxy consent decisions. The second extract was unusual in that this mother had made a conscious decision to allow her child to give blood for research, but not for the creation of immortalized cell lines. None of the other parents refused to allow this process on the basis that it was, in their opinion, a decision for their child to make when they were old enough to do so. When parents did refuse to consent to this process it related to their own fears and concerns and not about their ability or 'right' to make such a decision on behalf of their child. By illustrating the views of participants about the long term use of data generally and genetic databases in particular we can see that a number of issues emerge as relevant. These include: anonymity, confidentiality, consent and notions of risk. All of these concepts inform the context within which the collection and long term use of genetic and non-genetic information takes place.

Consent and decision-making – who is in control?

Issues of consent and decision-making within the research process were, for the child participants, connected to their experiences of taking part in the larger ALSPAC study. Because the children were recruited into the ALSPAC study, in most cases, prior to their birth or when they were very young children, it was important to establish how the children perceived the process of consent and decision-making. On the whole they perceived consent as a progressive relationship between themselves and their parents in conjunction with the researchers and others.

Participant: It would probably be shared with parents and children to see how different they think.
Interviewer: Okay about, so if the parents said no but you said yes what would happen then do you think?
Participant: They'll probably ask lots of other children and their parents as well, see what they think.
Interviewer: But then say they said oh I know we need to ask every child if we can use their, say they took a little bit of everybody's fingernail . . . Do you think you should decide whether they can do it or do you think mummy should decide whether they can do it?
Participant: Um, well probably you should decide first so if mum says yes and I say no they can't really do it 'cause I said no and it'll be my fingernail but if mum says no and I said yes I could probably convince her, but it would probably be sort of shared.

(Female child aged 10)

This extract is interesting as it demonstrates this child's perceptions of the decision-making process between children and their parents as well as illustrating an understanding of wider democratic decision processes. In this example the child explores the idea that consent might be agreed upon by the population as a whole, namely a consensus of views from the ALSPAC population. This child also makes a very interesting point that if her mother said yes and she said no, the study could not use her fingernails because they are her fingernails and not her mother's. This raises further questions about ownership and notions of gift relationships (see Tutton, this volume). So, can a parent consent to give a gift of their child's biological and non-biological material? Children perceive that tissues (in this case fingernails) belong to them. Within a legal framework they do not and cannot own biological material, but does that mean that another, in this case one with rights of proxy, has the right to give them away? Does it make a difference if we perceive ownership and thus gift relating to the body, or as described by Hilary Rose (2001) as information about the body? These questions will be re-addressed shortly.

We also found this child's exceptional comment about being able to persuade her parents to allow her to take part particularly interesting. Most children discussed joint decision-making but were not explicit in how they might persuade parents to change their minds and thus get their own way. Parents on the other hand gave such responses very frequently. They were confident in most cases that they had the ability to persuade children to their way of thinking as the following extract from a participating ALSPAC mother illustrates.

Participant: Well, I wouldn't break his arm and twist it and say 'you gonna definitely do it' but I would say 'it's for a very good cause and I want you to do it' and then he would probably say 'yeah' anyway.
Interviewer: What if he still said no?
Participant: He wouldn't [laughter].
Interviewer: OK.
Participant: Mother's last word.
Interviewer: OK, that's fine.
Participant: He'd do it and that's it.

(ALSPAC mother)

In relation to control and decision-making it is important to acknowledge the differential power relations that exist between individuals both within wider society and individual families. Childhood is a culturally and historically specific concept which has, in some instances, resulted in children being relatively powerless within existing legal and social frameworks (Oakley 1994). As these extracts illustrate however, the way in which this power is negotiated by children and parents is complex.

Priscilla Alderson (2002) addresses the position of children within bioethics and suggests that 'bioethics protects adults in ways which fail children' (Alderson 2002: 9). Discussing the way in which the 'protective ethic of respect for autonomy' of adults and children differs she suggests that 'informed and voluntary consent is left to parents, whose interests and values may conflict with the child's'(Alderson 2002: 9). The result of such a situation is, according to Alderson, that 'children may then be used as means to other people's ends without their willing consent' (Alderson 2002: 9).

Although in most cases parents felt that they would be able to explain to children why they 'should' take part in research which benefited others, they also made a clear distinction, which mirrors that currently enshrined in law (Huxtable 2000), between research on healthy subjects, and that related to treatment.

Participant: I said 'Well we'll go along, we'll see and if you don't want to do
it, you don't have to do it. But it would be really nice if you could
do it.'
Interviewer: Right, OK. But in terms of if it was treatment?
Participant: If it was treatment that was critical to his health, then, I think
he'd have to have it done.

(ALSPAC mother)

The law and guidelines for researchers currently differentiates between
treatment and research. The original Declaration of Helsinki does not allow
non-therapeutic research on non-consenting subjects, thus removing (legally
defined incompetent) children as potential research participants (World
Medical Association 1964). Generally, the guidance suggests that in relation
to research with children it should not take place unless the child benefits.
How this benefit is interpreted however does differ. The revised version of
the Declaration of Helsinki 'no longer requires that children or incompetent
research participants be the direct beneficiaries of the research, but rather
that such research be necessary to promote the health of the population
represented' (Knoppers *et al.* 2002: 222). In relation to treatment, the legal
position in the UK is that competent minors (individuals under the age of
18 who are able to satisfy specific competence criteria) can consent to treatment, even where parents refuse, but cannot refuse treatment if it is deemed
appropriate by medical personnel alongside parents or the courts (Huxtable
2000).

The result of this distinction is that within a treatment context at least,
the legal position of (competent) children to refuse treatment is curtailed,
yet this would not be enforced in a research context. If children are not
informed about when they are and are not allowed to share and make decisions,
this is potentially confusing and may undermine children's participation
in the process. For example, if a child was engaged in the decision-making
process about medical treatment, yet their decision to dissent was overridden,
this could influence how they view their role in other decision-making contexts.
The majority of children within the EPEG project talked about shared
decision-making. This suggests that they might not wish at this point to make
decisions on their own, they do however express views which suggest they are
beginning to assert their own agency in this context.

Interviewer: Yeah, so who would they, who could they write to then to see if
they could use the information?
Participant: The children.
Interviewer: Yeah.
Participant: I don't think it would be parents because it's the children who
filled in the forms.

(Female child aged 11)

This extract is problematic as although the children have filled in forms about themselves, parents have also released information about their children. Whilst the information contained might relate to the child, because it is completed by the parent further issues of consent and proxy consent are raised. In addition, children themselves are giving information relating to family life to researchers. For example information about sibling relationships and bullying:

Participant: Well it said in one question 'does your family spend a lot of time with you' and I put like in the middle and I thought my mum would get a bit offended about that, and they said 'is your family ever mean to you' and it was like 'never' or 'sometimes' or 'often' or 'all the time' and I put 'sometimes' because my dad can get a bit too stressed out and my mum can get a bit stressed out and my sister she's really bossy so she's, she like orders me around.

Interviewer: Right, yeah, so you didn't show that one to your mum?

Participant: No 'cause I know she'll get a bit upset about it.

Interviewer: Yeah, that's very thoughtful of you isn't it to hang on to it? Did you want to tell her?

Participant: I just think its better if I don't tell my mum.

Interviewer: Yeah okay, and do you think it's good that with some of the things 'Children of the 90s' put you can just keep between yourself and 'Children of the 90s', do you think that's good?

Participant: Well sometimes I feel a bit uncomfortable about writing it because I never really met many people from 'Children of the 90s' and they've never met me really so its kind of like talking to a complete stranger about life.

(Female child aged 9)

In relation to familial information collected for research, the case of Richard Curtin is particularly relevant. Curtin is a father who objected to the inclusion in research of his twin daughter and son, who had been enrolled in a research project based at Virginia Commonwealth University. The study requested information about other members of the 'subject's' family, in this case the twins' father. Curtin objected to the disclosure of familial information to a third party (the research team) on the grounds that his daughter giving information about him was an invasion of his privacy (Mathews 2000). In that particular case it was agreed that the university had 'violated Curtin's rights by not seeking his consent before sending a questionnaire that asked for personal information about him' (Mathews 2000: B7). In the case of children whose parents are giving proxy consent, a similar issue is raised when considering the long term use of information.

Researchers such as Mark Connolly and Judith Ennew (1996), and Roger Hart (1997) have all examined the concept of 'child centred research' and the implications of this notion on the way decisions in research are made. Summarizing their work Priscilla Alderson (2001) states:

> The lowest levels are the pretence of shared work: manipulation, decoration and tokenism. The next levels which involve actual participation are: children being assigned to tasks but at least also being informed about them; children being consulted and informed; and adults imitating but also sharing decisions with children. The top two levels are projects more fully initiated and directed by children.
>
> (Alderson 2001: 145)

Alderson and Jonathan Montgomery (1996) identify four stages of participation in shared decision-making. These included: being informed, expressing a view, influencing the decision-making and being the main decider. Children in the EPEG project when discussing shared decision-making remind us that these stages are not linear, but fluid. In different contexts, different levels of 'sharedness' will be achieved. In the case of children's involvement in treatment decisions for example, parents, where possible, are keen that children are being informed, but not if they perceive that this would unduly worry or concern the child. The result, according to Alderson, is that 'children are extra vulnerable when, as well documented by childhood studies, their own views and feelings and time are taken less seriously than adults' views and time' (Alderson 2002: 9). Within research, parents considered children to be the main decider, with themselves as parents influencing the decision-making. However, this appears not to be the way in which children themselves perceived the process.

The concept of proxy consent in research includes within it an understanding that children of this age (9–11) should assent or dissent to their own participation (Coughlin and Beauchamp 1996). In order to explore this further we examined the way in which children experienced specific activities and measures within the research process. On the whole the children found these tests interesting and fun to take part in. However, several children described incidents when although they felt unhappy or embarrassed to complete an activity or assessment, they did not feel able to refuse to participate. Some of these children felt that they were powerless to change what was happening to them, while for others to participate or not was a difficult choice to make.

Interviewer: So would you feel you could say no if you didn't feel like doing something?
Participant: I'd just be too shy really so I'd say yeah OK.

(Female child aged 10)

Differentiations between types of information and associated risks will be addressed shortly. However, this example illustrates the role of assent and/or dissent in the proxy consent process. Whilst many parents are clear that in a research context, as opposed to a treatment situation, they would not force their child to take part, those who believed in the value of the research also thought that they could 'persuade' their child to participate. As we have illustrated from the extracts earlier, children negotiate decision-making between themselves and others as an ongoing process. Children's positions in these negotiations change as they are given more power to make decisions, and are given more information on which to base them. The children's expectation to be given more choice and control over their involvement in the future has implications for the future provision of information to the children and their families for informed consent decisions. It is worthy of note that although the children already know that they can say no to any activity, the reality of their experience is that dissenting is difficult (especially in the context of physical one-to-one, face-to-face interactions). Such conflict suggests that children perceive adults' decisions as more powerful in this context than their own, emphasizing the importance of creating an accepting, non-pressurizing environment, to enable children to have a real choice about participation (Alderson 1995, Morrow and Richards 1996). Creating the conditions necessary to enable children to express their views, reflects the basic human needs and rights of the child in any research context (UN Convention of the Rights of the Child 1989, World Medical Association 1964) and in relation to genetic research in particular (Knoppers *et al.* 2002).

Parental consent to the long term use of their children's biological and genetic information

Both ethical and legal questions arose when we compared parent and children's responses to questions about the long term use of genetic and non-genetic information in non-therapeutic research. Children in particular, as was illustrated above, took the view that if another hypothetical study (Children of the 2000s or 2010s) wanted to use their data that they themselves should be asked. It is also evident from discussing these issues with children that their role in proxy decision-making is changing and will continue to change as they become increasingly 'competent minors' and young adults.[5] This view of increasing the role of child participants is consistent with the views of Steven Coughlin and Tom Beauchamp (1996) who suggest that 'to maintain confidentiality in minimal-risk epidemiological research, it is proposed that parental permission be waived and that mature minors be allowed independent decision making' (Coughlin and Beauchamp 1996: 215). Parents raised concerns about the long term use of information and, like the children, felt that any changes in the direction of the research or its purpose should be discussed with them and additional consent obtained.

Participant: I'm more cautious about that because I have some idea of what
happens nowadays, but if that's stored and in 50 years time you
could, somebody could do something wrong, y'know bad with it,
then I would be more cautious about giving permission for my
child's genetic information to be stored, protecting them.

(ALSPAC mother)

This extract relates to the long term use of information within a single study
context. Other issues were raised when discussing the use of information
for other purposes (different databases or for insurance purposes), or by other
researchers. The concerns raised here related to anonymity, continued consent
and potential use. With regard to the inclusion of children's data and information, the issue of anonymity raises further questions if, in the process of
protecting individuals' anonymity, the ability to withdraw from research at a
later date is curtailed.

Ownership was raised by child participants in the previous section. There
are a number of legal and ethical issues which arise in relation to the status
of information and biological samples 'given' within a research context (see
Tutton this volume). For example, is information about a child, provided by
a parent, the property of the child, the parent or the study it has been given
to? Does it make a difference if the information relates to the feeding habits
of a baby compared with information about puberty or adolescence? If a mother
agrees to the retention of placental tissue for research purposes, is genetic
information obtained from it the property of the mother, the child or the study?
Does it make a difference if it is genetic or non-genetic information?

Legally, perceiving the status of the child as fixed is problematic. Given
that parents have the right to consent on behalf of their children (alongside
the responsibility of doing so) it could be argued that the act of 'proxy giving'
is, in itself, unproblematic. However, in this context time is an important
variable as the time lag between giving and use could call into question the
rights of parents. It is possible that material 'given' by parents on behalf
of their child may be used after the role of proxy has expired. It is reasonable
to question therefore whether additional consent is required from the child
themselves either prospectively or retrospectively once they are of an age legally
to consent on their own behalf. Likewise, just as the differentiation between
the rights of children and parents to refuse treatment illustrates, we enter
a legal quagmire if a child was to refuse, for example, the use of genetic
information derived from placental tissue once they are an adult themselves.
We ask these questions because the responses we received from parents about
the long term use of data and the status of their own consent, let alone that of
their child, suggest that the process is complex:

Participant: That would be different then, I suppose my assumption about
the five years was that was what you are signing up for and you

can keep it for five years, and after that you have to throw it away, I think if, I think it would be unethical if people are under the assumption that you throw stuff away after five years and actually you kept it, it reminds me a bit about the Alder Hey Children's hospital, the children's organs that were being taken without the parents' knowledge, so I think there is a question there about the longevity of what you understand that material to remain in existence for, whether or not you trust the doctor after five years, if you [are] under the assumption that after five years it is gone, that should be it. So I think your example is almost like the person knows it is there forever but assumes that after five years you would be re-contacted, so that is the way I would have thought.

(Non-ALSPAC parent)

Whilst this view of active participation and consent was more prevalent than those adult participants who advocated a more traditional notion of 'gift' (see Tutton this volume), this could very well relate to the relationship which exists between adult participants and the particular study in which they are involved.[6] In relation to children, parents' concerns about the use of their own information over time, and the need for ongoing consent would further suggest that children too be given the ability to make decisions at a later date about information relating to them.

Even if we move outside of the realms of genetic material, the 'rights' of parents to give permission for the long term use of non-genetic informa-tion can be called into question. The rights of family members to disclose information about other family members, within a research context, was raised earlier (Mathews 2000). Whilst that particular case centred around whether a child could give 'private' information about a parent, the 'rights' of parents to give 'private' information about their children could become problematic in relation to the long term nature of longitudinal epidemiological research. Within the role of proxy consent, parents are able to give permission both for their own participation and that of their children. As such they are also in control of whether they consent to information, both genetic and non-genetic, about their child being given by them. The question we wish to raise, however, is whether a child would have the right, once legally competent, to challenge the 'giving of this gift'?

Paul Martin and Jane Kaye (1999), in an examination of the use of biological databases and medical records, found that the general view in the United Kingdom is that when ethics committee approval has been given, consent is not required when research is using anonymized personal information which does not harm the individual (Martin and Kaye 1999: 24). With regard to the inclusion of children's personal medical information within the Icelandic database, Martin and Kaye (1999) found that parents were given the option to refuse the inclusion of their children's material, yet, if this was not done, and the information was included, it could not be withdrawn at a later date. Indeed, there appears from other sources to have emerged confusion about the rights of children (and others) to later withdraw their data from the Icelandic database.

> The legislation offered citizens the right to opt out by mid-June 1999 . . . protected their right to opt out later; however, the law does not say whether they can withdraw their data . . . When the Council of Europe's Steering Committee on Bioethics asked the Icelandic Government whether data could be withdrawn, the official reply was that this was 'subject to negotiation'. However this claim has to be set against the record of the debate in the Althing where the Minister and Government supporters had explicitly stated that data once entered could not be withdrawn.
>
> (Rose 2001: 22)

Hilary Rose (2001) uses the Icelandic case as an illustration of the ethical issues involved in collecting genetic material for use in a database. Rose specifically identifies children as raising problems for the deCODE Icelandic project by claiming that 'the disenfranchisement of the children troubled [her] most' (Rose 2001: 25). Discussing the details of the ability of citizens to 'opt-out' of the Icelandic Health Sector Database she refers to the position of children as an 'arbitrary destruction of children's rights' (Rose 2001: 25). This is despite the fact that 'opinion polls indicate rather less enthusiasm [for the database] among the young' (Rose 2001: 12). Of particular relevance to children, it was acknowledged in Iceland that individuals could at a later date request that additional information was not included within the database, but again previously included data could not be removed. This suggests that once information has been given children do not have a right to the future withdrawal of that information from research even when the data might be stored and used in the future. Martin and Kaye suggest that the level of consent needed for the use of tissue samples and personal information in research is unclear. Furthermore they identify that whilst common law protects individuals in terms of the process of 'taking' the sample, similar individual control is not evident in the sample's subsequent use: 'in contrast, legislation allows individuals to control what happens to parts of their body and consent is required for subsequent use' (Martin and Kaye 1999: 48).

The legal framework within which the long term use of information is contextualized is both contradictory and problematic. It is exactly the difficulty with the proxy decision to 'give' or 'take' samples which raises issues about collecting such information from children. From children's own perspectives they see decision-making processes as an ongoing exchange of power between themselves and their parents. They believe that they should have an active role, either now or at a later date, in decisions about the use of information they have given. In terms of ownership and 'proxy gifting' we believe that all efforts should be made to include children's views prospectively in the long term use of data and information which relates to them.

Children's perceptions of personal information

Finally, in relation to proxy consent and the role of children in the collection of material for long term use in research, children also differentiated between the kinds of information which they may or may not agree to be used in the future. Central to the legal and ethical protection of child participants are the concepts of benefit and harm. Again these issues were explored in detail within the adult interviews, but will not be addressed here (Williamson *et al.* 2003). As was mentioned briefly earlier the notion of minimal harm is central to the ability of researchers to recruit children within non-therapeutic research. When discussing the future use of information children considered personal information to be particularly sensitive.

Participant: I think I should be asked if they had like personal stuff that they were looking at, I think I should be asked about that.
Interviewer: And what would, say, so, bring it a bit closer to you now, say that was happening and they had asked you, what would you say?
Participant: um, if it was really personal stuff I would probably say no, but if it wasn't that personal I would say yes.

(Male child aged 10)

Parents' views of what constitutes 'personal' information varies, and differs from that which children identified. It is assumed that because children's moral and cognitive reasoning develops over the life course, as young children, they are in need of paternalistic protection. However, protecting children from risks and harms which they may not yet fully appreciate does not explain why the concerns which children do identify are not taken seriously:

Although completing questionnaires or answering questions about one's conduct or personal relationships may not be disturbing, answering some questions, particularly for adolescents, may cause emotional distress. Young people, with their growing wish for self-determination, are particularly sensitive to infringements of privacy, and may strongly object to others learning particulars about their personal lives or behaviour. Loss of control over such information, whether through compelled disclosure or breach of confidentiality, subjects many young individuals to embarrassment and degradation.

(Coughlin and Beauchamp 1996: 209)

Given the methodological framework of the EPEG project and the growing body of literature about the rights of children to influence and shape their own life worlds, (Oakley 1994, Alldred and Edwards 1999, Alderson 2000, Neale 2002) traditional assertions about proxy consent which ignore the views of children are problematic. As we can see from the children's extracts above, children's concerns about the types of information which they consider more personal and thus sensitive are valid. They have concerns about personal information, the use of which could be embarrassing or uncomfortable. None of the parents who were interviewed suggested that their child's views of what was personal information might differ from their own, despite being asked for their views on different types of genetic and non-genetic information and being prompted to explain further what personal information might be.

Parents identified financial information, medical history, contact details, illegal activities and sexual behaviour as potentially sensitive or personal information. In some cases this was raised in relation to the types of information they have given over the years to the ALSPAC study. In relation to children, however, parents did not consider how their children might feel about answering certain questions. Children identified personal or private information as information relating to being hurt, bullying, friendships, family relationships, whether their parents were still together, problems at school, feelings and emotions, weight and body image and antisocial behaviour. Whilst children's views of what sensitive information is might change over time, partly on account of developmental changes and cultural expectations, the lack of recognition that children's views would be different, yet valid, we believe further questions the role of parents in the proxy consent process. Is it acceptable that the role of proxy consent appears to protect children from harm they might not identify at the expense of recognizing the harm that is important to them now? Whilst individual children grow into adults, as representatives of that group their views are important for the 'rights' of future children in that particular developmental phase. By including them in the decision-making processes of research, the views of participants can be included and addressed.

Conclusion

Many of the questions that have been raised in this chapter relate to the roles that parents, children, researchers and other governing bodies play in the protection of child research participants. The protective nature of this ethical framework has inherent within it assumptions about the relative positions of children and adults/parents within it which we need to acknowledge. The legal position of children with regard to the biological and non-biological samples which they have 'given', or have been 'given' on their behalf, is ambiguous. The questions which this ambiguity raises at present remain unaddressed. Children's situation with regard to consenting to the long term use of information about them is different to that of adults. We are not suggesting that children should be making their own decisions about participation alone, as many of the children we spoke to relied on the shared nature of this process. However, children's views are important in ensuring that their own concerns and interests are addressed both when they are children and when they themselves become adults. Essentially we are suggesting that the mechanism by which children participate in research which involves the long term use of biological and non-biological information needs to recognize the ways in which children might be excluded from a protective framework intended to protect them. As this chapter has illustrated this has a number of implications for participating children and their parents.

Specifically, we found that children currently underestimate the amount of control that they have with regard to their participation in non-therapeutic research. Unlike treatment situations parents would not 'force' their children to take part in non-therapeutic research, although they did believe that children could, and in some cases should, be persuaded. Children on the other hand, whilst they know they can say no, found this difficult on occasions. In this respect the setting in which children make decisions is important as is the information they are given about the boundaries and limits of their own control. For example, if children understand that there are certain decisions they are not allowed to make, then they should also be aware when decisions are in their control.

Second, we questioned the 'right' of parents to consent to the long term use of their children's biological and genetic information. The very notion of parental rights to make decisions within a proxy consent framework is, we believe, made problematic by the transitory nature of childhood when discussing the long term use of biological samples.[7] Finally, we have illustrated how parents and children's views of what is personal information differed. The majority of parents did not consider what their child might perceive to be sensitive information. This has implications for the validity of the proxy consent process if its aim is to ensure the protection of the best interests of the child. In this example, whilst the future best interests of the child may be being served by the parent in a paternalistic role, the current best interests of the child are not because their views are not incorporated within the current process. As this chapter has discussed, the many questions which have been raised are not adequately dealt with within the current legal framework where the position of children renders them relatively powerless in comparison with adult proxy decision-makers. In addition it has been suggested that 'adult-centric bioethics' (Alderson 2002: 10) fails to incorporate children and children's viewpoints adequately within its ethical frameworks. As such, concepts such as 'best interests' are located in opposition to notions of autonomy rather than enabling both parents' and children's perspectives to be included. All of these problems are exacerbated when we are discussing the long term use of children's information in databases because children become adults and as such their relative power and position change. This chapter has demonstrated that children have clear views and opinions about their experiences of participating in longitudinal epidemiological research. From these accounts we can observe children claiming a role in the decision-making process. It is our conclusion that by asking children about ethics and genetic research, this project has sought to include within the current ethical, legal and social debates about genetic research the views of those who, it could be argued, have the most to gain or lose from the current scientific endeavour.

Acknowledgements

The authors would like to thank the Wellcome Trust who funded this research (grant no. RJ3536), the project advisory group, and those children and parents who participated in the EPEG project.

Notes

1. The term 'pregnancies' rather than women is used here as some women were recruited into the ALSPAC study more than once in relation to different pregnancies.
2. These are know as focus@ sessions. The focus@ sessions are half day visits to the ALSPAC study where children complete a range of physical, psychosocial and biological tests. Online. Available HTTP: <www.ALSPAC.Bristol.ac.uk> for more information.
3. 'The Discovery Club' is an interactive club which participating children can join. They are sent newsletters and educational information. For more information about the discovery club see
   http://www.alspac.bris.ac.uk/Discovery/discovfrt.html 2003.
4. For a more comprehensive list of ALSPAC funders see
   http://www.alspac.bris.ac.uk/alspacext/MainProtocol/Section_12/12.2-12.4.htm
   #Funding_sources
5. The legal distinction currently made with regard to children's ability to make treatment decisions differentiates between competent and incompetent minors (Huxtable 2000).
6. The ALSPAC study maintains contact with participants over a long period of time and participation and consent are therefore continuous. These views may well differ if the study's contact with participants is less frequent or on a one-off basis.
7. In addition, but not discussed in this chapter, is the work of Alderson (2002) where she discusses the impact of genetic research on prenatal services and thus on specific groups of children and/or neonates.

References

Alderson, P. (2000). *Young Children's Rights: Exploring Beliefs, Attitudes, Principles and Practice*, London: Save the children/Jessica Kingsley.

Alderson, P. (2001). 'Research by children', *International Journal of Social Research Methodology* 4: 139–153.

Alderson, P. (2002). 'Utopia or dystopia? The new genetics as an environment for childhood', in M. Gollop and J. McCormack (eds) *Children and Young People's Environments*, Dunedin: Children's Issues Centre.

Alderson, P. and Montgomery, J. (1996). *Health Care Choices: Making Decisions with Children*, London: Institute for Public Policy Research.

Alldred, P. and Edwards, R. (1999). 'Children and young people's views of social research', *Childhood* 6: 261–281.

ALSPAC (2002). Online. Available HTTP: <http://www.ALSPAC.bris.ac.uk>.

ALSPAC (2003a). Online. Available HTTP: <http://www.alspac.bris.ac.uk/ALSPACext/MainProtocol/section4.htm> (accessed 24th June 2003).

ALSPAC (2003b). Online. Available HTTP: <http://www.alspac.bris.ac.uk/ALSPACext/MainProtocol/Section_8/8.4%20part%201.htm#Collection_of_biological_samples> (accessed 24th June 2003).

Connolly, M. and Ennew, J. (eds) (1996). 'Children out of place: Special issue on working and street children', *Childhood* 3 (2).

Coughlin, S.S. and Beauchamp, T.L. (1996). *Ethics and Epidemiology*, New York: Oxford University Press.

ELSPAC (2003a). Online. Available HTTP: <http://www.alspac.bris.ac.uk/elspac/protocol/chapters/E_protocol_chapone.htm#one> (accessed June 2003).

ELSPAC (2003b). Online. Available HTTP: <http://www.ich.bris.ac.uk/elspac/protocol/chapters/e_protocol_chapeight.htm>.

Golding, J., Pembrey, M., Jones, R. and ALSPAC team (2001). 'ALSPAC – The Avon Longitudinal Study of Parents and Children 1. Study Methodology', *Paediatric and Perinatal Epidemiology* 15: 74–87.

Goodenough, T., Williamson, E., Kent, J. and Ashcroft, R. (2003). 'What did you think about that? Researching children's perceptions of participation in a longitudinal genetic epidemiological study', *Children and Society* 17: 113–125.

Hart, R. (1997). *Children's Participation*, London: Earthscan/UNICEF.

Huxtable, R. (2000). 'Re M (Medical Treatment: Consent): Time to remove the "flak jacket"?' *Child and Family Law Quarterly* 12: 83–88.

Knoppers, B.M., Avard, D., Cardinal, G. and Glass, K.C. (2002). 'Children and incompetent adults in genetic research: consent and safeguards', *Nature* 3 (March): 221–224.

Martin, P. and Kaye, J. (1999). *The Use of Biological Sample Collections and Personal Medical Information in Human Genetics Research*, London: The Wellcome Trust.

Mathews, J. (2000). 'Father's complaints shut down research: U.S. agencies act on privacy concerns'. *Washington Post*, 12 January, p. B7.

Morrow, V. and Richards, M. (1996). 'The ethics of social research with children: an overview', *Children and Society* 10: 90–105.

Neale, B. (2002). 'Dialogues with children: children, divorce and citizenship', *Childhood* 9: 455–475.

Oakley, A. (1994). 'Women and children first and last: parallels and differences between children's and women's studies', in B. Mayall (ed.) *Children's Childhoods: Observed and Experienced*, London: Falmer Press.

Rose, H. (2001). *The Commodification of Bioinformation: The Icelandic Health Sector Database*. London: The Wellcome Trust.

United Nations (1989). *Convention on the Rights of the Child*, Geneva: UN.

Williamson, E., Goodenough, T., Kent, J. and Ashcroft, R. (2001). EPEG project: interim report,
http://www.bristol.ac.uk/Depts/Ethics/CEM/epeg_interim_report.htm

Williamson, E., Goodenough, T., Kent, J. and Ashcroft, R. (2002). 'Ethical protection in epidemiological genetic research: participants perspectives, (EPEG project): preliminary findings', paper presented at BSA conference, Leicester.

Williamson, E., Goodenough, T., Kent, J. and Ashcroft, R. (2003). 'Genetic epidemiological research: participants' perspectives on "drawing the line"', *Who Twists the Helix?* Conference paper, 16–19 March 2003.

World Medical Association (1964). *Declaration of Helsinki*, World Medical Association.

Chapter 9

'Public consent' or 'scientific citizenship'?

What counts as public participation in population-based DNA collections?

Sue Weldon

Introduction

Informed consent is at the heart of ethical practice in medical research, but recent involvement of research participants in clinical genetics has led to a suggestion that this is inadequate as an ethical basis for participation (see, for instance, Chadwick 2001, Chadwick and Berg 2001). Here it is argued that public participation in genetic databases is both an ethical and a wider social issue. Informed consent does have an important (even symbolically crucial) role to play in addressing ethical research practice for individual participants. But, rather than extending the notion of consent to increasingly wider groups of people, it is being suggested here that there is a need to think in terms of different kinds of participative relationships between science and society. It is important to realize that individuals encounter, and participate, in medical research within a social context and they engage at many levels. This implies a wider concept of engagement and another level of participation based on 'scientific citizenship'.

This chapter examines the setting up and use of DNA population 'biobanks', from the perspective of the public consultation about their ethical implications and social impact. A UK House of Lords Select Committee report (2001) on the collection of human genetic databases has emphasized the challenges posed by their development for the way medical research is practised (House of Lords 2001). These challenges relate to international concerns about potential invasion of privacy, commercial exploitation and the difficulty of obtaining fully informed consent from participants. Consultation carried out by the Medical Research Council (MRC) also addresses another key challenge for policy-makers relating to public acceptance of the genetic research.[1] For instance, in the wake of a number of recent health-service scandals, declining public confidence in the governance of medical research has been noted.[2] It has been suggested that an essential component in reversing this trend is to ensure that there is widespread public involvement in any new research proposals. Paul Martin and Jane Kaye (2000) make the point that 'without widespread public support for population genetic studies there is a real danger that human genetics could become the next biotechnology scare' (Martin and Kaye 2000: 1148).

So far there is very little detailed information about how these challenges can be addressed in a socially responsible manner. It is important to know *who* will get a say, in what *manner* and to what *effect*. Whilst there is a long tradition of public participation in medical research, many people argue that involvement in genetic research has special implications, not only for those individuals who participate but for the future of society in general. There are many who point out that ethical concerns cannot adequately be addressed by the notion of participation of consenting *individuals*. Wider ethical frameworks need to be posited on ideas of citizen participation and donation to *society*. Indeed, there are persuasive arguments that individual rights need to be weighed against our social duty to promote the common good (Chadwick and Berg 2001). But a crucial concern relates to public acceptance of genetic research trajectories, in that the public expects not only to know what is going on but also to be given an opportunity at the outset to negotiate what counts as the 'common good'.

Although many of the implications of biomedical research have been conveniently separated out into the domain of bioethics, which deals with ethical principles underlying individualist issues such as informed consent, confidentiality and privacy, conventional bioethics has had little to say about wider social concerns. These concerns include not only issues specifically about the forms of governance established to regulate the proposed research and about whether people really trust the institutions controlling the initiatives, but also about the direction the research is taking. In the context of public engagement in addressing these concerns Peter Healey (2001) has described it as 'the social equivalent of informed consent'.[3] However, it is not clear whether and how it would be possible to extend the notion of consent to society as a whole. Would it be a form of 'public consent' – a popular vote for instance? If not what would be a more appropriate form of public engagement? For instance, it has been suggested that – in a participatory democracy – citizen participation should extend to determining the uses of these population databases and the extent of commercial involvement. It could be argued that, in a participatory democracy, citizen participation might go even further than consenting to, or accepting, an already prescribed research agenda and that there is a role for citizens in negotiating alternative healthcare futures in which the 'new genetics' is one of a number of alternative research paradigms.

The chapter draws on various academic strands of social science research. More specifically, it is informed by current findings from an ongoing comparative study of the social, ethical and legal implications of population-based databases in the UK, Iceland, Estonia and Sweden (ELSAGEN). The study aims to anticipate and address a whole range of questions raised by these genomics research initiatives. Part of the study draws on empirical social research to determine public perceptions of the ethical implications of these new technologies. This specific research objective is to provide knowledge about the implications of human genetic databases for governance and democracy. Partners from the four countries will be comparing quantitative and qualitative data relating to public perceptions of privacy and trust in the institutions governing these new initiatives. Another aspect of the study compares the way protocols are being negotiated, particularly in relation to public consultation. For instance, it is very interesting to see how the approach taken in the UK, in setting up UK Biobank, compares with (and has been informed by) the debates happening in other countries, as for instance the controversy about plans to set up an Icelandic Health Sector Database (HSD).

These plans to establish an Icelandic HSD[4] have been set in motion by the State in collaboration with a commercial enterprise deCODE Genetics who have claimed that public acceptance has been obtained and that the arrangements are the product of the democratic process (Zoega and Anderson 1999). The culmination of this process of 'collective acceptance' is a Parliamentary Bill passed in 1998. However, in the opinion of many critics viewing these negotiations from outside the country, it could be argued that Icelandic people are having their individual rights overruled in favour of public benefits – only to see their genetic inheritance converted to a 'privatized' and subsequently tradable commodity (see, for example, Rose 2001). In contrast, the negotiations surrounding the UK Biobank (and in the aftermath of the 'Great GM debate' in the UK and recent medical research scandals) have been particularly attentive to the role of public participation in determining suitable guidelines for acceptable informed consent practices, and to protect individual privacy. There has been ongoing concern (mediated by the strategic oversight of the government's advisory body the Human Genetics Commission – HGC 2000) to promote an open and informed public debate about benefits and possible commercial abuses of DNA databases. A key question that this chapter addresses is whether, or to what extent, this wider involvement could count as 'public consent' and if not whether it would be more appropriate to regard it as a form of 'scientific citizenship'.

Participation in biobanks

Medical research has always relied to some extent on collected and stored data and the forthcoming UK Biobank project purports to be 'the world's biggest study of the role of nature and nurture in health and disease' (Wellcome Trust/MRC 2002). It promises to use information from the study to develop improved diagnostic tools and targeted therapies for the common diseases that affect people in later life. But it is important to begin by looking at some of the factors informing this international drive to establish large-scale genetic databases. It appears that the current research need for population-based DNA databases has arisen out of, and is seen as a natural progression of, the human genome mapping project. As the Director of the Wellcome Trust – Mike Dexter – has put it: 'The UK Biobank is a natural progression of the [Wellcome] Trust's involvement in the Human Genome Project'[5]. The House of Lords report on 'Human Genetic Databases' (2001) endorses the benefits outlined by the project partners in stating that a database of this nature: 'has the potential for making a major contribution to healthcare and the development of new treatments' and could build on the unique reservoir of information provided by the UK's National Health Service (House of Lords Select Committee on Science and Technology 2001: 8). The report goes on to make the point that, although the mapping of the human genome could be described as a revolutionary scientific achievement, the knowledge will be of no practical use in isolation. In the wake of gene sequencing the public benefits will flow only when we move from simple description of our genetic makeup to explaining how it acts. In the future we need to understand the *functioning* of genes in different environments. For such projects a great deal of personal information is required – including genealogical data, personal lifestyle information and knowledge about the environmental context – and public participation is crucial in achieving that aim.

It is recognized that one of the features of a venture such as this is the need to set up new regulatory frameworks to establish the rights and obligations of research participants or donors. It has also been argued, by MP Ian Gibson, that this is such an important and unprecedented initiative that it requires prior 'parliamentary scrutiny and a wider public debate' (Gibson 2002).

In the UK, in Europe and the rest of the world advances in genetics are now subject to layers of statutory and advisory control that are in constant flux. The collection and use of personal genetic information raises particular concern in relation to a range of social, legal and ethical issues that have been identified by the MRC (2000) after much discussion with ethicists, lawyers and interest groups. The ethical use of personal genetic information has also been one of the main concerns of the House of Lords report, and has been the subject of a wider ranging investigation conducted by the Human Genetics Commission. Overall, a number of issues were considered to be significant. In addition to informed consent, these included confidentiality, commercial interests, ownership, access and feedback. Confidentiality has always been central to our doctor–patient relationship in the UK. It is the basis for the high level of trust that patients place in healthcare professionals to maintain privacy. Particular concerns arise in the case of DNA samples, where information contained on a database can have implications for a donor's family or for the donor's future prospects. Commercial involvement and use of the data collections warrants special consideration in relation to commodification and 'privatization' (through patenting for instance) of information that many people argue should be maintained in the public domain. It follows that ownership is a particularly pertinent issue, where commercial interests apply. Access to a sample collection by outside agencies, such as other research bodies and the private sector, can also create conflicts of interest. Confidentiality and consent arrangements may be compromised if the data are transferred with access to the key to identification. In the UK, access by third parties to databases is determined by the requirements of the Data Protection Act (1998). In setting up a database it is considered to be important to be aware that patients have a right to have feedback on information that affects their interests (even though they may choose not to exercise that right). Feedback may be viewed as an essential element of ongoing consultation. DNA samples are again a special case because of the implications for relatives, insurance, mortgage loans and in situations where participants can be identified. All of which highlight the importance for anonymization of the data.

Policy advisors have taken the position that the need to obtain individual informed consent from donors is paramount. Where the data are to be stored and used for 'secondary' purposes, i.e. other than for one specifically identified purpose (and where the data are in any way identifiable), consent arrangements are more complex. In particular it would not be possible to inform a research subject of the risks and benefits of the research and the wider social consequences. One way to address this issue would be to ask for 'broad' (rather than narrow) consent.[6] The MRC guidelines suggest that, if possible, information should be given about the type of studies the sample may be used for.

The role of individual informed consent

In medical practice informed consent is a very special consideration, to the extent that there is a higher standard of informed consent in clinical and/ or medical research than is required by common law. It has traditionally been viewed as the basis upon which an ethical relationship between an individual clinician/researcher and a patient/donor can be negotiated. In that context bioethicists have pointed to a role that is not only of practical, but also of symbolic value in both protecting and respecting the individual participant (Chadwick and Berg 2001). A recent Department of Health report, the UK Research Governance Framework (2001) sets out the terms for informed consent explicitly by stating that: 'all studies must have appropriate arrangements for obtaining consent and the ethics review process must pay particular attention to those arrangements' (DoH 2001: paragraph 2.2.3). This is also a fundamental consideration for ethical practice worldwide. The World Medical Association (WMA) revised the Declaration of Helsinki in October 2000 for the fifth time to emphasize in much clearer terms than ever before the duty that doctors owe to research participants. In terms of informed consent it says that each potential subject must be adequately informed of the aims, methods, sources of funding, any possible conflicts of interest, institutional affiliations of the researcher and the anticipated benefits and risks of the study. Contrary to this in the Icelandic case the manner of obtaining participant's assumed consent, by allowing them to 'opt out', has been described as a complete reversal of the standard demanded. The Declaration of Helsinki states that the subject should be informed of the right to abstain from participation, or to withdraw from the study at any time, whereas, as the Icelandic case indicates, once a record has been added to the database complete removal may be problematic. These two consent issues of the Icelandic study illustrate some of the more controversial aspects of the proposal which have led to international criticism.[7]

As we have seen the principle of informed consent is very well described and expectations of good practice in DNA biobanks are high. Nevertheless, there is still a great deal of concern about how this can actually be achieved because many bioethicists argue that genetic research raises significant problems for consenting arrangements, not least of these being the wider social implications of the research, uncertainty about where the research might lead and the need to safeguard the proper and secure use of all the knowledge that this kind of database would generate. Bioethicist Ruth Chadwick has questioned the adequacy of a traditional view of informed consent in genetics research (Chadwick 2001). She points out that it is an ethical principle that relies too heavily on individuals to make a decision about issues which not only affect their own interests but also those of a wider constituency. There is a need to balance the rights of the individual research participants against social benefits (and disbenefits) arising from the research. Yet another aspect to consider is whether it is reasonable to expect people to consent to donate samples and to accept any responsibility for their involvement in research that would not benefit them directly. The projected longer term benefit arising from research using databases includes a new paradigm for healthcare in which diagnosis and treatment of disease could be revolutionalized by the knowledge about the genetic basis for those diseases. In announcing the go-ahead for the UK Biobank in 2002, Professor Sir George Radda, Chief Executive of the UK Medical Research Council, suggested that: 'in 20 years time we may see individualized approaches to disease prevention and treatment' and that: 'it may be possible for a GP to prescribe drugs and other treatments designed specifically for people's own make-up'.[8] This is an optimistic view of the future which makes no reference to any possible adverse consequences. Even so, projections such as this raise questions about who would be the main bene-ficiaries of this smart healthcare. Pharmaceutical stakeholders would certainly stand to gain from these developments, but population databases will not necessarily directly benefit the individuals who supply the samples since the research is conducted over a long period. Even with benefit-sharing practices, such as those suggested by the Human Genome Organisation's statement (2001)[9] which proposes a more equitable solution in which pharmaceutical companies distribute a proportion of their income for public healthcare research, and to developing countries for humanitarian aid, it could be very difficult to decide which specific people would be eligible to share benefits. Benefits (and disbenefits) arising from the research have to be thought of as accruing to a wider community. These problems with individual informed consent in genetic research have been discussed in great detail by Chadwick, who argues that:

> The potential for harm appears to be significant not only to individual subjects but also to groups of which they form a part. The nature of the harm tends to be associated with the use of and access to information.
>
> (Chadwick 2001: 209)

It has been argued that different mechanisms may be required to address these two sectors of society (see for instance Chadwick and Berg 2001). In genetics all information supplied has implications for other family members in terms of inherited conditions and genetic pre-dispositions. But there is also an issue about wider communities with inherited tendencies (Weijer 1999). One example, is where particular mutations have been identified through studies of Ashkenazi Jews. Should we, for instance, be seeking community consent if the research is used to characterize ethnic groups? This is based on a potentially misleading understanding of genetic conditions that could reify differences between ethnic groups and lead to a version of community consent in which community is defined in genetic terms that ignores how these diseases are actually also found across other ethnic groups.

In a country as ethnically and culturally diverse as the UK, it is very difficult to define communities. In some situations they may be seen as 'aggregated individuals'. For instance, single issue groups, such as those with an interest in finding tests, therapies and eventual cures for specific genetic conditions (such as cystic fibrosis and thalassaemia) are likely to have a different, and perhaps more 'consumer-oriented', attitude to the use and sharing of information than members of the wider public, who may be more concerned about longer term consequences and risks to society as a whole. There are wider social benefits and consequences to consider in establishing a population-based genetics database and in using it for research purposes. Information arising from the database could be used in any of a number of ways that may require negotiation about their impact and acceptability for a wider public. Extended access to information and sharing of data, commercialization and privatization of information arising from the database are examples of consequences that could be construed in either positive or negative ways. It is clear therefore that a balance needs to be struck between individual (or aggregated individual) rights and concerns and those of society. But it is not clear whether these concerns can be addressed by widening a notion of informed consent (that has traditionally been based on a one-to-one researcher–participant relationship) from the individual level to community, or wider public, level within a framework of individual choice?

The need to establish a more workable ethical framework, within which these wide ranging and conflicting interests can be resolved, has led the Human

Genetics Commission (HGC) to identify what they believe to be over-arching basic principles relevant to personal genetic information and designed to promote 'social interest – or the common good' (HGC 2002: 38). Their advisory report on 'Balancing interests in the use of personal genetic data' suggests that genetic knowledge may bring people into a special moral relationship with one another – one that might be seen as a form of solidarity (HGC 2002: 38). They suggest that a principle of solidarity, accompanied by the concept of altruism – and echoing the concept of solidarity in the UNESCO Universal Declaration – be based on the assumption that we all share the same basic human genome. The key features of these concerns were for the most part identified as affecting individuals. Crucially, however, the report makes a strong case for a genetic citizenship, in arguing that it is important to see the individual as a member of society with an active role in promoting wider social interests. In this context, but still within a framework of individual informed consent, a duty is projected on participant donors to act in their capacity as citizens, in addition to and at the same time as exercising their individual rights and responsibilities. This is a move that acknowledges the wider context but fails to recognize that there appears to be little opportunity at present for participants to influence the wider issues. Where is the opportunity, for instance, to participate as a citizen in deciding the fate of the database or the direction of research – or even in deciding whether to invest public money in this particular kind of population-based database? One might argue that, given the complexity of the issues and the level of concern mentioned earlier, these are aspects that should be opened up for political scrutiny and public debate and should subsequently become part of the research protocol.

Setting up the protocol and consulting the public about the UK Biobank

The following section looks at the ways in which these wider public concerns and 'ethical' issues have actually been addressed in setting up the protocol for the UK Biobank. From a social science perspective it is always significant to reflect on where the boundaries are drawn, how public participation is construed and how concerns are elicited and interpreted. It is clear, for instance, that public consultation is not an unmediated form of participation. As many analysts of public participation point out, it would be a mistake to imagine that 'the public' is anything other than intrinsically heterogeneous and any claim to have consulted the public begs the questions 'which publics', 'in what capacity', and 'at what level'? Aside from the fact that public consultation can be conducted at many stages in a research trajectory there are issues about the kinds of interactions that are happening, the quality of the dialogue and the status of the knowledge exchanged between consultant and consulted.

From its inception in 1999, the UK Biobank partners emphasized the need to work within an ethical framework. The key ethical principles in their approach to the study included continuous consultation with all stakeholders (from patients to healthcare professionals), obtaining informed consent, holding the information in public ownership and for public benefit and granting no exclusive access by any one commercial company (unlike the much criticized Icelandic database). It is also claimed that the views of the public, health professionals, scientists, non-government organizations and industry obtained as a result of consultation studies will be taken account of. A workshop held in 2001 to develop the protocol for UK Biobank reported that the gaining of participants' informed consent is 'both desirable and necessary'[10] in the way Biobank is organized and run, but emphasized a shift in expectation by the public such that: 'more explicit consent should be sought than had been the case in previous medical research studies'. Significantly this was reported as part of a movement from viewing participants as 'research subjects' to 'citizens' (MRC/DoH/Wellcome Trust 2001).

Public consultation was commissioned by the project co-ordinators (Wellcome Trust/MRC 2000 and 2002) and by the HGC (2001) to discover the range of public concern in relation to current advances in medical genomics generally, and more specifically in relation to the setting up of UK Biobank. In the UK these consultations have included both quantitative surveys[11] and qualitative focus groups.[12] In addition to public consultation, both the UK government's House of Lords Select Committee on Science and Technology (2001) and the Parliamentary Office of Science and Technology (POST 2002) conducted their own investigations about the opportunities and challenges arising from the use of genetic databases. Alongside this, an ethical framework was developed in consultation with a number of other interest groups, including scientists, social scientists, ethicists, lawyers, health professionals, patient groups and civil society groups. A range of ethical issues were identified, including: the nature and scope of consent; the relationship between UK Biobank and other research groups in respect of confidentiality; issues around anonymization of the data; the relationship between UK Biobank and commercial interests; and the role of an oversight body and its relationship with the existing research governance framework.

The report of an ethics workshop held in 2002 emphasized the central role of consent in creating an ethical framework for participant recruitment:

> The debates continually return to consent as the most fundamental of all issues. Recruitment into the study would only be successful if the Biobank participants had confidence in the UK Biobank's procedures for ensuring that appropriate and ethically sound procedures for consent, confidentiality and the regulation of commercial access to samples and data were in place.
>
> (The Wellcome Trust/MRC/DoH: 2002)

Can these consultations count as consent?

The consultation processes outlined above emphasize a stated commitment by UK Biobank partners to an unprecedented and participatory level of consultation and dialogue with wider stakeholders. Individual consent emerges for them as the key to ethical conduct. Nevertheless, and in spite of all this, the POST report argued that the project raised a number of important issues that had received relatively little scrutiny at *parliamentary* level (POST 2002). The report also suggested that several NGOs (Human Genetics Alert, Consumer's Association and GeneWatch UK) would like to see more consultation to address *public* concerns about issues of consent, confidentiality and ownership before the project starts recruiting. Overall, the MRC/Wellcome Trust and HGC surveys reported that there was broad support for Biobank and enthusiastic acknowledgement that developments had the potential to offer valuable opportunities to treat and cure many diseases. The majority of people appeared to have responded to questions about consent by endorsing its central role in obtaining information and storing it on databases. However, against this, the call for parliamentary-level scrutiny and wider public debate emphasized a requirement for wider negotiation about a regulatory framework, within which a project like UK Biobank would operate, and the need to get this framework right at the outset. This was an issue that was made clear when the Chair of the House of Commons Select Committee on Science and Technology (Ian Gibson MP) raised it during a parliamentary adjournment debate in July 2002:

> The project needs to be conducted and organised by experts, but such an important and unprecedented step must not be taken without parliamentary scrutiny and a wider public debate.
>
> (Gibson, Hansard 3 July 2002)

Separating ethical concerns from scientific issues

However, policy concerns at this level, about the need for input into the framing of the project, are as much about the broader research framing and the scientific methodology as they are about the ethics of individual consent. For instance, a question was raised about the problems that might be encountered in combining (qualitative and context dependent) lifestyle information with 'hard data' obtained from DNA sampling. The implications for healthcare policy were that this method of sampling could: 'skew towards over-emphasizing the genetic influence on disease processes because it is the only thing on which Biobank will provide hard data' (Gibson, Hansard 3 July 2002).

None the less, it was clear from a subsequent parliamentary scrutiny of the MRC by the House of Commons Select Committee on Science and Technology carried out in December 2002 how the development of the scientific protocol had been addressed separately, and distanced conceptually, from the ethical framework. In answer to a question put by a member of the Select Committee to the MRC about the adequacy of the consultation process, as we see, consultation/participation of the public was confined only to contributing to the development of the ethical framework:

MP: Has the public consultation influenced the creation of the protocols for Biobank so far?

MRC: I think probably the answer to that is that the protocols, as we have them, is actually the scientific protocols . . . it is largely scientific at this stage. The ethical issues have been carried out in parallel with all that . . .[13]

The point being made here is that, in developing the protocols for the project, 'objective' scientific protocols are conceptually (and physically) separated from more 'subjective' debates about ethical issues. Two assumptions are being made. The first is that the scientific development of the protocol is immune from ethical considerations, defined apart from areas requiring public partici-pation and therefore not an area for input from the public or an area where matters of public judgement or evaluation are relevant. The second assumption is that ethical considerations apply only at the level of consent.

The significance of making these assumptions about public participation might be better understood from an entirely different perspective. The 1999 GM controversy has been a salutary lesson in how to misinterpret public concern about issues of science policy. In the strength of feeling it generated in the UK, the public debate about the GM issue caught many policy-makers unawares and subsequently resulted in changes within the framework of governance for biotechnology. As a direct result of this upheaval and public disquiet, two new commissions (the Agriculture and Environment Biotech-nology Commission and the Human Genetics Commission) were created, partly for the purpose of consulting and engaging in debate with citizens about the future of biotechnology innovation in Britain. This whole new emphasis on citizen engagement was captured subsequently by a House of Lords report on Science and Society (2002) in the following way in stating that:

Direct dialogue with the public should move from being an optional add-on to science-based policy making and to the activities of research organisations and learned institutions, and should become an integral part of the process.

(House of Lords 2000 para. 5.48)

It could be argued that the controversy about GM biotechnology has very little relevance for public policy and ethical oversight of the 'new genetics'.

Although the evidence from research into public perceptions of biotechnology has indicated that research and development in medical genetics is looked on more favourably than GM technology, this is not, as has often been supposed, based predominantly on individual self-interested assessment of personal risks and benefits.[14] Other factors play a more important part in the discrepancy – such as belief that in this area of biotechnology there is stricter regulation and risk assessment and better access to information through trusted professional intermediaries – general practitioners (GPs). This insight is significant because it now appears that science-based innovation and strategies continue to be based on the misconceived but entrenched view that projects public concern as individually self-interested, subjective and intellectually vacuous. Brian Wynne (2001) has raised this point in relation to recognition of a general crisis of confidence in science, but more specifically in relation to a relatively recent focus on the need to address the 'ethical' aspects of these new technologies. Wynne has argued that a renewed focus on ethics as a distinctly separate aspect of the debate has helped to maintain an unhelpful distinction between the scientific and ethical aspects of science-based policies. This subsequently leads to the assumption that ethical practice requires the public to be engaged in negotiation of the latter (more 'subjective') aspects of the development of the technology, but not the former. 'In this way, public concerns about the purposes, driving forces and conditions of innovation research can be deleted and misunderstood as exaggerated and irrational concerns' (Wynne 2001: 476).

Thus the development of the protocol guidelines for the UK Biobank has been undertaken in good faith against a background of a changing policy agenda, towards a more participatory style of governance, and taking into account public concern about what are considered to be 'ethical issues'. But it is argued here that consultation carried out so far has still 'framed out' parliamentary and public concerns about broader, and also in some sense, *scientific* issues. In doing so it fails to address participation at the level of what will be referred to as 'scientific citizenship'.

Public consent or scientific citizenship?

So far I have looked at participation in biobanks from a perspective that invites extension of the concept of individual consent, within the context of negotiations with donors, to take account of wider social issues in addressing the balance to be struck between individual rights and duties and those of society as a whole. Given that any notion of 'public consent' would have to be wider than that given by single interest groups or 'aggregated individuals', it is important to ask how 'the citizen' can be addressed within this context (as the HGC report advises) without additional levels of participation? For instance, do we need to superimpose a wider public debate about the framing of the issues? If this is required for adequate public participation would the outcome of a wider social and ethical debate somehow 'trump' individual informed consent? Charles Weijer (1999), for instance, notes an asymmetry in that social acceptance of a research project need not overrule an individual's right to refuse to participate, but social lack of acceptance could overrule an individual's right to opt in.

Given the amount of attention that has already been given to individual informed consent, how and at what level would wider social concerns be negotiated? It seems clear that this needs to be applied 'up stream', for instance, as we noted, at a strategic policy level in negotiating regulatory frameworks and conditions under which research priorities might be judged. The question then arises as to whether this 'up stream' negotiation could still be framed as a form of public consent? For instance, if it amounts to a simple choice of whether to accept or reject a proposal – even applied 'up stream' – there is no sense of agency for people to negotiate or debate the issues (about what counts as *the common good*'). Public consent is what the Icelandic government seem to be claiming when they announced that the result of a democratic process of public debate was the public acceptance of (or consent to) the Icelandic Health Sector Database – in the form of a Parliamentary Bill.

In examining the question of what counts as public participation there is a need to examine certain assumptions about how the participation processes are framed, how the public is construed and how consent or acceptance is construed. Is the information about the research framework and the scientific knowledge being accepted uncritically? It is generally accepted as a principle of active citizenship in a democratic society that people must be able to influence policy decisions that affect their lives. Alan Petersen and Robin Bunton (2002) are cautious, however, about an uncritical use of 'active citizenship' in public forum discussions about genetics and its public health benefits that are dominated by experts. Many of the decisions about the funding of high tech issues like biotechnology and genetics seem to require highly specialized knowledge, and the public is often portrayed as lacking in the ability to appreciate fully the complexity of the science. Alan Irwin (1995) considers the possibility for a more active *scientific* citizenship in negotiating the part played by science and scientific expertise in our everyday lives. Citizen concerns, he argues, need to be seen against a background of technical development issues: 'which go beyond matters of *application* and into the very fabric of science as a knowledge system' (Irwin 1995: 105). This is part of what has been described as 'a new move for dialogue' – in the UK at least. In a climate where public confidence in science, and policy based on science has been eroded in recent years a shift is taking place to the point at which: 'today's public expects not merely to know what is going on but to be consulted' (House of Lords Select Committee on Science and Technology 2000: para. 5.1).

I began by quoting Healey's comment, made in the context of a move towards democratization of science (in the aftermath of the GM debate), that this requirement could be seen as 'the social equivalent of informed consent'.

But in today's democratic society citizenship is envisaged as more 'active' than mere passive consent. As research into public perceptions of GM food has indicated, citizens need opportunities to negotiate meanings (see for instance the evidence given in the PABE report – Marris *et al.* 2001). These insights extend to public views about what sorts of health agendas should be supported, what counts as a significant risk etc. The inevitable conclusion is that people do not want to be fed a pre-framed set of issues to *consent* to, as passive citizens. Informed consent arises out of a particular context that constructs participation in a particular way (originally consent to a particular individual medical intervention). In that sense it operates within a specific understanding of people and science and does not address participation at the level of active citizenship. Informed consent has normally been applied 'down stream' where the only choice – even if it is informed – is whether to consent or not and where there is no dimension of collective democratic negotiation, of the nature of the decision or the direction of the innovation path. Irwin suggests the need to look more critically at particular participatory initiatives (for instance in technology assessment) to see how they address the public and the 'scientific citizen'.

Engaging at citizen level

In the following section I outline recent moves towards a more participatory style of engagement, but noting the need to examine this move with the same critical eye that has so far been applied to informed consent. I have argued in this chapter that public participation in genetic databases is both an ethical and a wider social requirement. Although informed consent does have an important role to play in addressing ethical research practice for individual participants – and even for patient and consumer groups – there are issues about scientific citizenship that are being framed out and cannot therefore be negotiated within the dual notions of information-giving and individual consent. Equally, it is impossible to refer to active citizenship, or even *scientific* citizenship, as if the terms of engagement are fixed. For instance, we need to define which public is being addressed. The public can be many things: individual patients, clients or consumers; single interest groups; community groups; or citizens of the nation state (or the European Union), and they engage at many levels.

I made the point earlier that there is now a widespread consensus, at policy level, that science's relationship with the public is in a critical phase. Increasingly, and in all areas of public policy, notions of active citizenship and public participation are taking over from the representative mode of governance (see for instance, Marinetto 2003). In what has been described as: 'a new mood for dialogue' between scientists and the public,[15] investments are being made by research councils and policy bodies in piloting innovative and participatory modes of consultation and processes of dialogue (including surveys, focus groups, citizen juries and consensus conferences). There is now an accumulated body of experience in the UK and in other countries about these new forms of participation.

In evaluating what has now become known as 'participatory technology assessment' (pTA), Simon Joss and Sergio Bellucci (2002) refer to the need for socially legitimate decision-making in a climate of uncertainty, diversity and often contested values. They provide a number of justifications: first that in a democratic society it could be seen as a 'right' to participate (however indirectly). But there are stronger reasons than that. When it ensures participation by those who are directly, and indirectly, affected by the research the assessment takes on a new dimension based on richer knowledge and understanding of the issues. In the new spirit of open dialogue it also addresses inequality of access to a policy world that has traditionally been closed and elitist. Finally, the optimist view is that participatory engagement can help to create better outcomes by providing an arena where potential controversy can be resolved (or cooled down) and new avenues explored. Overall, it is hoped that this will contribute to more ethically and politically accountable research outcomes.

Public participation in scientific and technical projects, in its broadest sense, requires citizen involvement in the processes of policy and decision-making at national level, and by a wide range of 'publics' (including stakeholders). The aims and types of practice vary from 'constructive technology assessment' (which integrates the views of users into research trajectories) to the promotion of wider public and political debate as a contribution to public policy-making. Participation can operate at many different levels. Sherry Arnstein developed a classic model to define levels of public consultation and citizen participation (Arnstein 1971). A 'ladder of participation' represented levels ranging from *informing* the public through to *involving* the public and, at the highest level to citizen *empowerment*. The ladder was designed to help practitioners understand the concepts of participation and active empowerment, but it was also a normative tool (in inviting practitioners to move up the ladder). This brief explanation illustrates the need to be reflexive about the level at which people are being invited to participate and the social and political context in which the consultation/dialogue operates.

I have referred to a range of new forms of citizen engagement and intimated that they should not be used uncritically. Modes of participation, at whatever level, need to be critically evaluated according to the relationship between participant and researcher and the context. The argument is that participatory 'tools' to promote engagement and dialogue with the public (such as surveys, focus groups, stakeholder workshops, citizen juries, consensus conferences) need to be evaluated according to their ability to afford 'civic agency'. Irwin (2001) points out that different models adopt different approaches to 'the public' and to scientific citizenship. For instance, he looks at the quantitative survey market research model as a 'customer-responsive mode' that presents a 'passive scientific citizen' as opposed to a more active and empowered citizen at the deliberative democracy level of a citizens' jury.

Closer evaluation of the citizens' jury model, which is upheld by Irwin as a more participatory approach to citizen engagement, illustrates a further aspect of the question: 'what counts as participation?' The question is: can the participatory process acquire legitimacy with decision-makers to the extent that it actually makes some impact on decisions? In an evaluation of a pilot citizens' jury, carried out in Wales, Peter Glasner and David Dunkerley questioned the effectiveness of a process that ritually separates the scientist from the citizen and leaves the lay citizen 'seated at the ringside of the decision-making process' (Glasner and Dunkerley 1999: 323). I have also made the point, in tracing the process of developing the Biobank protocols, that it would be wise to be cautious about allocating the status of citizenship to participants (as if that guaranteed effective entitlement to influence ethical conduct in research).

Turner (2001) makes a distinction between passive and active citizenship. He is sceptical about the granting of citizen entitlements in contemporary global and 'high tech' societies and suggests that it is more valuable to see it as a process of *acquiring* active agency through participation (Turner 2001). Turner argues that this would not have been quite so problematic in more traditional contexts, when citizen rights were framed in such a way as to protect individuals within a (relatively local) marketplace. However, within the context of a modern 'globalized' economy and high-risk society (cf. Beck 1992), and for these new rights and obligations to be enacted effectively, we need new and revised forms of governance. The implications of transnational commercial exploitation of science – for instance in moves towards patenting aspects of the Human Genome – have already led to considerable public concern about how genomics can be governed at a level over and above the national (or even European) level. It was this concern that promoted John Sulston (formerly the Director of the Sanger Centre) to write:

> We in Western Society are going through a period of intensifying belief in private ownership, to the detriment of the public good. Through a process of globalization these beliefs are being inflicted on the world as a whole – and not just via companies: as nations too, we are unable to make sensible collective decisions when the only rules we know for bargaining are those of competitive greed.
>
> (Sulston and Ferry 2002: 278)

The notion of participation based on active citizenship is dependent on one further set of conditions, arising this time from the ability of research establishments to enter into dialogue and debate and not to misunderstand the genuine concerns of the wider public. As I explained earlier, much consultation has already been carried out on behalf of Biobank partners to ascertain public perceptions of genomics and to identify concerns which people have about how genetic information is used. The key to active public agency appears to lie in the quality of the engagement – based on genuine two-way understanding – and in the appropriate use of the results in determining policy and developing protocols. This assertion can be backed up by political reality, as I have noted.[16]

Conclusion

The question: 'what counts as participation in population-based DNA collections?' has been addressed through examination of the limitations of informed consent and the possibility of active scientific citizenship. Traditional approaches to informed consent have addressed citizens as individual passive citizens with individual subjective concerns – in effect as consumers – given a choice whether to accept a participant role or not. This is not considered by anyone to be an adequate answer to the issues raised in setting up population-based collections of genetic and medical data for research purposes, the use of which may have far reaching social and ethical implications.

A challenge for policy-makers and regulators is in how to approach participants as citizens (with an obligation to promote the common good) rather than as passive research subjects. Real input into policy does not just come down to making individual choice about a branded product – a choice to take part, or not to take part, in UK Biobank. It is clear, from research into public perceptions of agricultural biotechnology, that many people operate within a wider context, seeing themselves as making choices as citizens, not just as consumers. But to do that they want to know not only if the product reflects their needs and is safe for them to use but also whether the brand is socially acceptable. This begs the question of how participants' citizen rights (their 'civic agency') can be respected. In searching for a better understanding of the issues I have explored the possibility of 'scientific citizenship' as a mode of engagement that builds on the desire for a better, more accountable and more participatory relationship between science and society. This is a cautious approach that acknowledges the very real problems of acquiring civic agency. In asking about the construction of the 'scientific citizen' in consultation – or in pTA – Irwin suggests that:

> The relationship between science and democracy should not be about a search for universal solutions and institutional fixes, but rather the development of an open and critical discussion between researchers, policy makers and citizens.
>
> (Irwin 2001: 17)

This is not a form of 'public consent' – about whether to accept or reject a set of market variables. Traditionally, the boundary between science and society has been policed by experts. But, in order for the lay public to participate fully in genetic research as citizens, the technologically optimistic view of medical research might need to be opened up so that citizens can find a role, alongside researchers and other professionals, in negotiating science's 'licence to practise'.

Acknowledgements

I gratefully acknowledge the insights and feedback on this chapter received from Ruth Chadwick and Mairi Levitt. The chapter also draws on work being carried out as part of the ELSAGEN project (Ethical, Legal and Social Aspects of Human Genetic Databases: A European Comparison) financed between 2002 and 2004 by the European Commission's 5th Framework Programme, Quality of Life (contract number QLG6-CT-2001-00062). However, the information provided is the sole responsibility of the author and does not represent the opinions of the aforementioned.

Notes

1. A programme of qualitative research to explore public perceptions relating to the collection of samples for research, carried out by Cragg Ross Dawson for MRC/Wellcome in 2000 (MRC/Wellcome Trust 2000).
2. In 1999 a public inquiry was held at the Alder Hey Hospital in Liverpool to investigate the removal of organs from dead children without parental consent. Also at this time, the deaths of 35 children under the care of heart specialists in Bristol led to an inquiry which severely criticized the standard of care given to the children. In 2000 Dr Harold Shipman, a general practitioner (GP) was convicted of murdering 15 of his patients (but the estimated figure could be over 250 patients). All of this has led to widespread media coverage and subsequent calls for more rigorous medical accountability.
3. Witness statement to House of Lords Select Committee on Science and Technology. Session 1999–2000 3rd report, 'Science and Society'.
4. The Icelandic Health Sector Database will include information taken from medical records and will be connected to two other database sources: one containing genealogical data and the other containing genetic information from biological samples supplied by donors.
5. Director of the Wellcome Trust in a news release. Recorded on the MRC website 'Biobank UK'. MRC (2002) 'The UK Biobank gets funding go-ahead'.
6. Broad consent is the term used by Chadwick and Berg (2001) to distinguish consent required for research on an unspecified range of conditions, rather than on one narrow specified range.
7. For further information about the controversies surrounding the Icelandic database see Arnason (2003).
8. Professor Sir George Radda in a news release. Recorded on the MRC website MRC (2002) 'The UK Biobank gets funding go-ahead'.
9. In the light of concerns about benefit sharing, the international Human Genome

Organisation's (HUGO) ethics committee made a statement in 2000 advocating wider Benefit Sharing.

10. MRC/DoH/The Wellcome Trust (2001). Report of the UK Population Biomedical Collection Protocol Development Workshop. Royal College of Physicians 17 April 2001.

11. For example a survey of 1249 people conducted by MORI for the Human Genetics Commission asked a total of 71 short questions about people's attitudes towards, and knowledge of, genetics.

12. For example a consultation for MRC/Wellcome, based on 16 focused group discussions about issues surrounding the collection and storage of personal genetic information.

13. Transcript of the House of Commons Select Committee scrutiny of the MRC. 4 December 2002.

14. Series of focus groups carried out in five EU countries, to determine public perceptions of agricultural biotechnology in Europe (PABE), reported this specific point (Marris *et al.* 2001).

15. House of Lords Select Committee on Science and Technology. Session 1999–2000 3rd Report, 'Science and Society'.

16. Further support for this crucial aspect of engagement is emerging from research into public perceptions of biobanks (currently being carried out for ELSAGEN), which is finding that people do not trust public agencies to listen to their concerns, and that they therefore feel no sense of 'agency' to act as citizens within current institutionalized participatory practices.

References

Arnason, G. (2003). 'Second thoughts on biobanks – the Iceland experience', in E. Einsiedel (ed.) *Crossing Over – Genomics in the Public Arena*, University of Calgary Press.

Arnstein, S. (1971). 'A ladder of participation in the USA', *Journal of the Royal Town Planning Institute*, April 176–182.

Beck, U. (1992). *Risk Society: Towards a New Modernity*, London: Sage.

Chadwick, R. (2001). 'Informed consent and genetic research', in L. Doyal and J. Tobias (eds) *Informed Consent in Medical Research*, London: BMJ Books.

Chadwick, R. and Berg, K. (2001). 'Solidarity and equity: new ethical framework for genetic databases', *Nature Review Genetics* 2: 318–321.

Cragg Ross Dawson (2000). *Qualitative Research to Explore Public Perceptions of Human Biological Samples*. A report for The Wellcome Trust and Medical Research Council, London.

Gibson, I. (2002) *Petition on 'Biobank', House of Commons Hansard Debates*, 3 July 2002. Online. Available HTTP: <http://www.publications.parliament.uk> (accessed 27 January 2004).

Glasner, P. and Dunkerley, D. (1999). 'The new genetics, public involvement, and citizens' juries: a Welsh case study', *Health, Risk and Society* 1: 313–324.

Healy, P. (2001) *Witness statement to House of Lords Select Committee on Science and Technology, Session 1999–2000, 3rd report*, Science and Society. Online. Available HTTP:
<http://www.parliament.the-stationery-office.co.uk> (accessed 27 January 2004).

House of Lords Select Committee on Science and Technology (2000). Session 1999–2000, 3rd report, *Science and Society*, London: The Stationery Office.

House of Lords Select Committee on Science and Technology (2001). Session 2000–01, 4th report, *Human Genetic Databases: Challenges and Opportunities*, London: The Stationery Office.

Human Genetics Commission (2001). *Public Attitudes to Human Genetic Information*. People's Panel Quantitative Study conducted for the HGC, London.

Human Genetics Commission (2002). *Inside Information: Balancing Interests in the Use of Personal Genetic Data*. A report by the HGC, London.

Irwin, A. (1995). *Citizen Science: A Sudy of People, Expertise and Sustainable Development*, London: Routledge.

Irwin, A. (2001). 'Framing the scientific citizen: science and democracy in the biosciences', *Public Understanding of Science* 10: pp. 1–18, London: Institute of Physics Publishing.

Joss, S. and Bellucci, S. (2003). *Participatory Technology Assessment: European Perspectives*, London: University of Westminster.

Marinetto, M. (2003). 'Who wants to be an active citizen? The politics and practice of community involvement', *Sociology* 37: 103–120.

Marris, C., Wynne, B., Simmons, P. and Weldon, S. (2001). *Public Perceptions of Agricultural Biotechnologies in Europe; Final report of the PABE research project*. Commission of the European Communities. Online. Available HTTP: <http://www.pabe.net> (accessed 4 December 2002).

Martin, P. and Kaye, J. (2000). The use of large biological sample collections in genetics research: issues for public policy', *New Genetics and Society* 19: 165–191.

Medical Research Council (2000). *Personal Information in Medical Research*, London: MRC.

Parliamentary Office of Science and Technology (POST) (2002). *The UK Biobank*, London: POST.

Petersen, A. and Bunton, R. (2002). *The New Genetics and the Public's Health*, London: Routledge.

Rose, H. (2001). *The Commodification of Bioinformation: The Icelandic Health Sector Database*, London: Wellcome Trust.

Sulston, J. and Ferry, G. (2002). *The Common Thread: a Story of Science, Politics, Ethics and the Human Genome*, London: Transworld.

Turner, B. (2001). 'The erosion of citizenship', *British Journal of Sociology* 52: 189–209.

Weijer, C. (1999). 'Protecting communities in research: philosophical and pragmatic challenges', *Cambridge Quarterly Healthcare Ethics* 8: 501–513.

The Wellcome Trust/MRC (2000). *Qualitative Research to Explore Public Perceptions of Human Biological Samples*, London: The Wellcome Trust.

The Wellcome Trust/MRC (2002). *Biobank UK: A Question of Trust: A consultation exploring and addressing questions of public trust*. A report conducted by People Science and Policy Ltd.

Wynne, B. (2001). 'Creating public alienation: expert cultures of risk and ethics on GMOs', *Science as Culture* 10: 4.

Zoega, T. and Anderson, B. (1999). *The Icelandic HDS: deCODE and the 'New Ethics'*, Proceedings of an International Conference, Tallin, Estonia.

Chapter 10

Tissue collection and the pharmaceutical industry

Investigating corporate biobanks

Graham Lewis

Introduction

The pharmaceutical industry is making increasing use of human genetic databases created by the integration of genetic data obtained from human biological material and other data, such as personal lifestyle and medical information, in order to study the relationship between genes and disease. This chapter examines the several methods that pharmaceutical companies use to access human tissue samples and related genetic information (commonly known as genetic databases) and assesses the size and extent of such activity. It also explores the reasons why the industry is interested in tissue collections and genetic information and why investment in human biological material and related bioinformatics products has been expanding dramatically and is likely to continue to do so.

Four models of pharmaceutical industry access are identified: 'in-house' collections established by drug companies themselves; the use of corporate intermediaries in the form of clinical genomics companies; collaborations with existing public collections, such as hospital pathology collections, and other, research-based, tissue banks; and industry use of newly built public collections incorporating public health records and other personal information, such as the UK Biobank, the Icelandic Health Sector Database and similar initiatives in other countries.

The second of these routes, access via clinical genomics companies, is the most significant at this point in time, apart from pharmaceutical companies' own internal efforts at building genetic databases, and the activities of a number of such companies are discussed. Two other important trends examined are the commercialization of existing public collections, often through academic–industry collaborations; and the creation of new national biobanks – large population-based collections that incorporate well-defined samples and related patient information obtained through healthcare delivery systems. The chapter concludes with a brief discussion of the policy issues raised by these various developments.

The chapter is premised on the belief that an understanding of industry involvement in the collection and manipulation of human biological material, part of what Dorothy Nelkin and Lori Andrews (1998) call the commercial-ization of the body in the age of biotechnology, is a highly significant aspect of the post-genomic era. Mention must be made of previous research on tissue commercialization, in particular work by Paul Martin and Jane Kaye (1999) on genetic databases for the Wellcome Trust and subsequent research (Martin 2000, 2001, Kaye and Martin 2000); and research by Jens Laage-Hellman (2001, 2003) directed at the relationship between public biobanks and clinical genomics companies in the Swedish context. This chapter endeavours to build upon, and extend, their efforts.

It should be noted at the outset that this is a difficult subject to investigate from a quantitative point of view. The pharmaceutical industry is notoriously secretive as regards its activities, and it has proved difficult to obtain hard information from individual companies regarding the extent and scale of tissue banking undertaken, and the size and composition of industry genetic data-bases, as this information is generally considered to be proprietary. An idea of the size and type of collections held by genomics companies is somewhat easier to obtain since such companies are in the business of marketing their tissue collections and associated data to the pharmaceutical industry, plus they are heavily engaged with venture capital markets. This means the business model and overall strategy adopted is generally more transparent. But the market for genetic information is intensely competitive, and the genomics industry has a well-earned reputation for hyperbole. Because of this, care must be taken to distinguish promotional claims from hard evidence as regards individual firm capabilities and the extent to which individual pharmaceutical companies rely on a particular source for tissue and genetic information.

The tissue collection and genetic database industry

Human biological samples are collected for a number of purposes in health-care systems, including diagnosis, monitoring treatment and, increasingly, for research. A tissue collection is a collection of such material either routinely sampled or collected for a specific purpose. Other terms commonly used to describe collections (all of which are used in this chapter) include tissue bank, tissue repository, DNA bank and biobank – with the latter term increasingly common when referring to large population-based collections, such as the UK Biobank and similar initiatives in other countries.

It is important to recognize that pharmaceutical industry investment in tissue banking, either through in-house collection or via other channels, is but one aspect of a very much larger tissue repository industry totalling many thousands of repositories that has been operating for many decades. Tissue specimens have been collected for at least 100 years and the scale of collection overall is huge. According to the US National Bioethics Advisory Commission (NBAC)[1] the total amount of stored human biological material in the US, as of 1999, was estimated to be more than 176 million individual samples; with over 282 million unique specimens, and with more than 20 million samples added each year (NBAC 1999). However, the proportion of these samples that reside within corporate databanks is unknown. Indeed, it is unlikely that these figures will include such samples and, since this time, the number of samples held by pharmaceutical and biotech companies has increased dramatically.

Most repositories are often long-standing collections directed at improving knowledge of specific disease states and providing suitable specimens for ongoing research by academic institutions and, in many cases, commercial organizations. Many collections are funded either directly or indirectly, by national governments or, in the case of the United States, the federal government. Tissue collections also vary considerably, ranging from formal repositories to the informal storage of blood or tissue specimens in a researcher's freezer. The size of US archives, for example, is estimated to range from less than 200 to more than 92 million specimens. The two largest tissue repositories in the world, the National Pathology Repository and the DNA Specimen Repository for Remains Identification, are housed in a single institute, the Armed Forces Institute of Pathology (AFIP), with more than 94 million specimens. Another very large repository is that at the US government-funded National Institutes of Health (NIH), with several million specimens (Eiseman and Haga 1999).

In 2001, DGI Inc., a US-based consultancy firm, announced its intention to collect information on potential corporate tissue databanks linked to population data, in the context of ethical responsibilities towards such samples (Jones 2001), but at the time of writing had yet to begin this work (Jones 2003). An overview of potential US sources is provided by the NBAC (NBAC 1999, Jones 2001) and by a RAND Institute report (Eiseman and Haga 1999). The vast majority of tissue in such collections was, and is, collected for diagnostic or therapeutic reasons, and not primarily for research, although it may be used for this purpose on occasions. However, several repositories have been established specifically for use in research. In addition, several very large longitudinal studies collect and bank samples from study participants, with the US NIH being particularly active. Likewise, a fair amount of research simultaneously creates tissue collections or contributes to tissue banks. Collectively, these contain several million specimens.

Besides collection for diagnostic purposes and use in research, tissues are also collected and stored for a variety of other reasons, typical examples being blood and organ banks, and DNA for forensic investigation and identification purposes. In most countries, sperm, ovum and embryo banks store specimens for anonymous donation or for later use by the individual storing the material. Umbilical cord blood banks also store blood for anonymous donation and later use by families banking their newborns' cord blood. Such developments are part of a long-term trend towards the commercialization of body tissue, a process that has been underway for many years. Biotechnology techniques have transformed a variety of human body tissue into valuable and marketable research materials and clinical products in recent years, as well as products and services in several other areas, including consumer products and the storage of blood prior to surgery or embryos during IVF (Nelkin and Andrews 1998). Tissue collection and the marketing and exchange of genetic data are also increasingly part of a global industry. It is however extremely difficult to gauge the scale of these activities.

Tissue banks are not only sources of physical tissue, however, but also genetic information in the form of databases and related digital information, such as microarray and gene expression data. This information may be combined with and incorporated into other types of information, like individual lifestyle information and personal medical records. Indeed, the primary interest of users of tissue banks for research purposes (as opposed to diagnosis or treatment) is the data that can be extracted from the tissue, not the biological material itself. Collections of such data are usually called genetic databases, a term that describes their main function, the storage of genetic data in a form that allows it to be organized, retrieved or mined in specific ways and for specific purposes over time, irrespective of the status of the sample from which it originated.

As Sonia Le Blis (2001) notes, depending on the context, genetic information can be considered as a material, a piece of information or a perception, yet genetic information is rarely given an explicit definition, as if its content were readily apparent and unequivocal. Yet the question needs to be asked as to whether such information refers only to the result of an analysis of a DNA sample, whether DNA itself should be considered genetic information, and whether clinical or family data can even be described in these terms.

All users of human tissue for genetic studies are confronted with issues to do with the collection, storage and use of that tissue – issues such as tissue quality, informed consent, and questions around 'ownership' and intellectual property rights (IPR). Yet as already noted, researchers, whether corporate or academic, are primarily interested in genetic data *derived from* tissue samples, not the tissue itself. Physical tissue and the genetic information derived from it, including data from other sources such as health and lifestyle information, is conceptualized as one and the same from the point of view of the discussion that follows, unless otherwise stated. Where a distinction is felt necessary, it is specifically noted.

Pharmaceutical companies and tissue collection

The demand for human biological resources and genetic information retrieved from them arises primarily from two research areas within the pharmaceutical industry. The first is the search for genes and biological markers that correlate with specific disease states (gene expression or functional genomics).

The second is the study of the relationship between individuals' genetic profile and drug response (pharmacogenetics) (see Corrigan this volume).[2] The first of these, drug discovery research involving gene expression and target validation, requires disease tissue (and non-disease controls), while pharmacogenetics research requires large numbers of individual DNA samples.

Both of these research areas potentially utilize genetic association studies, for which large population-based collections (biobanks) and related personal and environmental data are required.[3] In the next decade, tissue-based industrial research is likely to extend to other, more complex, areas of research, like proteomics,[4] tissue engineering[5] and stem cell research[6] – areas that are at present primarily of basic research, rather than commercial, interest.

Interest in the commercial possibilities of genetic databases derived from tissue samples has followed on from the international Human Genome Project (HGP). As many commentators have noted, the HGP was merely the beginning of a long process of further research involving the interpretation, elaboration and commercialization of the sequencing of the human genome – what Rose has termed the commodification of bioinformation (Rose 2001). Until the function of a particular gene and its role in pathology has been established, raw sequence information is of little value, and research to link gene sequences (genotypes) to biological function or diseases (phenotypes) is complex and time consuming. Due to the complexity of disease causation, this type of research requires large well-defined populations (Martin and Kaye 1999, Martin 2001).

Technically, studies identifying gene sequences involved in inherited disease can call upon powerful, well-established, mapping techniques to identify genetic changes in the form of polymorphisms (single nucleotide polymorphisms or SNPs being the most common) and other gene mutations and deletions associated with the pathology being studied. Despite the doubts of some commentators as to whether gene mapping studies and the search for complex traits in human populations will ultimately provide successful drug targets, the pharmaceutical and biotechnology industries are investing heavily in tissue banks and genetic information sources.

Powerful scientific arguments also support the use of models based on human tissue, rather than conventional animal-based models, for the biological screening of investigational new drugs and studies exploring drug action at the molecular level (Coleman 2003). Generally speaking, few animal species are sufficiently similar to humans to serve as a wholly reliable surrogate, although cost considerations and availability also play an important part in the choice of pharmacological model. The use of human tissue permits investigation of targets and/or the actions of test compounds in the target species, humans. This enables selection of the most effective targets (drug receptors) and the most efficacious and least toxic compounds at the earliest stage possible in the development process, thereby reducing the chances of failure in the clinic. Increases in drug development costs and decreasing returns from R&D

are therefore other factors driving tissue-based research, as the industry becomes increasingly focused on the inefficiencies of the R&D process and the 'target validation bottleneck' (Coleman and Clark 2003). The following sections review the scale and extent of corporate tissue collections and genetic databases, and provide examples of typical locations. As described in the introduction, corporate access to tissue supplies and genetic databases occurs in four ways: 'in-house' collection; access through licensing agreements or similar arrangements with clinical genomic companies (including dedicated tissue companies); access to existing, often publicly funded, collections such as those held by hospitals and pathology labs; and access to newly created population-based collections (biobanks). Most pharmaceutical companies use more than one of these channels to supply their various requirements for genetic resources. Also, whilst the activities of pharmaceutical companies are distinguished here from those of genomics firms, it should be noted that drug firms often invest in genomics companies as part of collaboration agreements. These investments can be for a variety of reasons: to ensure access to samples, or bioinformatics and proprietary technologies such as genotyping, or to buy expertise and 'know-how' in these fields.

While it is not possible to determine accurately the extent and scale of corporate banking activity, it is clear that the creation of large-scale tissue banks and associated genetic databases has expanded enormously during the past five years and can be expected to grow at a rapid rate in the future. Interview data collected from industry scientists and documentary evidence demonstrate that all the large pharmaceutical companies are engaged with the world of tissue banking and the collection of genetic information to some extent or another. In this sense, DNA information and access to biobanks can be viewed as the 'raw material' of the industry's future development.

As Martin and Kaye (1999) note, sources potentially available to commercial firms also include publicly funded research studies into the genetics of common diseases, family collections linked to genetic services, pathology specimens collected during routine work and samples provided by participants in clinical trials. The commercial exploitation of all of these sources has continued and expanded, with the last source in particular, samples from clinical trials, increasingly markedly as companies routinely collect and store samples during conventional drug development processes for possible future DNA analysis.

Here we have chosen to define tissue repositories according to ownership or location (e.g. public or private, internal or external). However, these resources may also be categorized according to access arrangements and the extent to which constraints are placed on use and, most important, identifiable links to donors (Wylie and Mineau 2003). Characterization in this fashion is also important because the extent to which genetic data can be related to individual donors establishes the value of that data.

Pharmaceutical industry collections

There are no published figures detailing the overall size, type and location of tissue banks owned by the pharmaceutical industry, although it is known that all the major pharmaceutical companies are collecting samples, either directly or through the use of clinical research organizations to collect and store samples. Evidence on tissue banking provided to the UK House of Lords, for example, provides an insight into industry activity, but it contains little quantitative detail and is now also out of date (House of Lords 2001).

The degree to which different companies engage in collection and storage of tissue and genetic data depends in part on company strategy towards genetics-based drug development. The maintenance of storage facilities and establishment of sophisticated computerized retrieval and informed consent procedures is both technically demanding and expensive. A company must have some idea of why it is investing in such systems and be prepared to make the substantial investment required to build and maintain such systems. Some companies, such as GlaxoSmithKline (GSK), have adopted a robust approach to genetics-based research generally by establishing a dedicated unit for genetics R&D that is able to intervene in development projects across the company to ensure strategic objectives are met. But even the more cautious companies, in terms of corporate perceptions and investment in the 'promise' of pharmacogenetics and other genetics-based drug development strategies, have adopted a 'just in case' approach to tissue banking, routinely storing samples in case they wish to retrieve genetic data from them in the future.

In the case of GSK, vigorous support for genetics research is reflected in the large tissue collections maintained by the company, which has built considerable expertise in handling such collections.[7] In addition, GSK have agreements granting access to samples and associated bioinformatics databases with several leading clinical genomics companies, including First Genetic Trust and Gene Logic (both discussed below). AstraZeneca, like other global pharmaceutical companies, is also investing heavily in genomics research, though to a lesser degree than GSK, with a policy of in-house collection through academic partners and clinical trials, and agreements with a number of genomics companies. As already noted, most companies are also routinely collecting samples from clinical trials. Other large pharma companies who have adopted such a policy besides GSK and AstraZeneca include Novartis, Roche, Pfizer, Bristol-Myers Squibb and Wyeth. These companies have also signed up with clinical genomics companies as part of their functional genomics and pharmacogenetics research programmes.[8]

Clinical trials consist of four main phases. In phase I, the drug is given to a small number of healthy volunteers for tolerability and dose studies. In phase II, a larger group of patients suffering from the target disorder is given the drug to demonstrate efficacy. A larger randomized clinical population is selected for efficacy studies in phase III. The data from these three phases form the basis upon which regulatory agencies decide whether or not to authorize sale of the drug. An additional phase, phase IV, occurs after approval is granted, to broaden knowledge of the product's actions and safety profile and possibly to extend indications. Collection of DNA samples from clinical trials involves patients undergoing treatment and therefore differs from methods discussed in other chapters (see Haimes and Whong-Barr, Busby, Williamson *et al.* this volume), since these focus on collection from healthy individuals only. Implementation of privacy legislation, such as the US Health Insurance Portability and Accountability Act of 1996, means that in some states the legal ramifications surrounding use of clinical trial samples remain unclear (Jones 2001). Similarly, there are a number of issues around the definition and interpretation of informed consent when clinical trial samples are collected for possible future use.[9]

Samples collected via clinical trials may be stored 'in-house' or they are archived by the contract research organization (CRO) undertaking the trial for the company. All major clinical trials providers, such as Quintiles, Covance, and PPD Development, have genomics capacity and are developing 'in-house' genetics research and clinical expertise as well as offering storage facilities for pharma companies. The industry's approach is summed up in the words of Novartis' head of pharmacogenetics: 'We now systematically collect DNA from every patient in every clinical trial, analyze that for variations and then at the end of the trial do association studies between genetic variation, efficacy and adverse effects' (Melton 2003: 923). The net result is that companies are collecting and genotyping many thousands of samples every day.

Clinical genomics companies

Another common method used to access human biological material and genetic databases is through clinical genomics companies. Access via this route may take various forms and vary over time depending on factors such as internal resources, research goals and overall company strategy towards genetics research and drug development. Commercial repositories – banks of tissue and data to serve the needs of the diagnostic, pharmaceutical and tissue engineering industry – are comparatively recent phenomena. An early example of pharmaceutical industry interest in this approach was SmithKline Beecham's US$125 million investment in Human Genome Sciences in 1993 – often considered the birth of the genomics industry (Laage-Hellman 2003). Since then, a large number of companies have been founded on the basis of selling information on disease genes (pharmacogenomics), and/or identifying the relationship between an individual's genotype, and in particular, single nucleotide polymorphisms, or the arrangement of these on the genome (haplotypes), and drug response (pharmacogenetics). Estimates put the market for tissue and related information to be worth between US$550 million and 5 billion (Stuart 2001).

The following outlines the business model adopted by a few selected clinical genomics companies and the types and size of tissue collection and genetic databases held by them. This is intended as a 'sampler' of the types of activities engaged in by such companies (which worldwide now total several hundred) as space limitations prevent a full account.[10]

The activities of First Genetic Trust (FGT) are specifically based on what the company believes to be one of the main obstacles for development of pharmacogenetics and personalized medicine: people's fear that companies will not keep personal genetic data safe. The company essentially acts as an intermediary between pharma industry researchers and patients, turning responsibility for informed consent and confidentiality over to a third party. Whether this arrangement will appeal to industry in the longer term remains to be seen. FGT claim that companies want to hand over responsibility, but evidence also suggests that companies are crucially aware of the importance of maintaining high standards and some may be reluctant to relinquish control. None the less, FGT is one of the leading genomics firms with several high profile collaborations, including GSK, Pfizer and the leading CRO, Quintiles.

FGT does not hold tissue itself but stores genetic information in its secure database and updates consent via the Internet when necessary, so that 'through our Internet-based systems . . . researchers can efficiently generate, manage, and analyze genetic and medical data'. For patients, the company promises 'a protected environment in which to maintain their privacy and the confidentiality of their genetic information while participating in genetic research'. For drug companies, another important recent development is the link with physician networks provided by companies like FGT, enabling direct access to many thousands of clinical trial patients/samples for pharmacogenetics programmes. For example, FGT is collaborating with Radiant Research, a Seattle-based site management organization (SMO) providing electronic access to clinical trial populations through physicians at 40 sites across the US (First Genetic Trust 2003).

Genomics Collaborative, Inc. (GCI), a major US-based genomics company, maintains a large-scale proprietary repository linked to detailed medical information collected from patients at over 400 sites worldwide. By 2003, the company had recruited over 115,000 patients and collections continue across a wide range of disease states. GCI applies high throughput genomic analysis, including SNP genotyping, DNA sequencing and microarray analysis, to samples for target discovery and validation purposes. Customers for GCI services include GSK, Millennium Pharmaceuticals, Merck, Pharmacia, Wyeth and Celera Diagnostics. GCI also offers commercial DNA and tissue banking services for collecting, processing and storage of biomaterials for industry, academia and governmental agencies, and is building a tissue bank for the government of Singapore.

Gene Logic is another leading US genomics company offering various proprietary gene expression databases derived from clinically important tissues.

Company sources say that all samples are rigorously collected and analysed, and data enhanced by powerful data mining and visualization tools. The cornerstone of Gene Logic's operations is the company's vast tissue biorepository of over 50 organ types, which the company sources from centres around the world. Like GCI, expression analysis is then performed on normal, diseased and treated tissues, for a range of diseases. Like Ardais (see below), Gene Logic's data processing systems are built in close collaboration with Affymetrix, the leading microarray platform company. Gene Logic has agreements with Roche, Schering-Plough, IDEC Pharmaceuticals, Fujisawa, Takeda and Mitsubishi Pharma, plus several other genomics companies.

The UK genomics company Pharmagene has collaboration agreements with several major pharmaceutical companies plus smaller biotech and drug discovery companies, including, Bayer, Bristol-Myers Squibb, Johnson & Johnson and Schering-Plough in the USA, and AstraZeneca, Boehringer Ingelheim, GSK, Janssen, Merck, Pfizer and Roche in Europe, plus several Japanese companies. The company has been collecting tissue for five years and employs a combination of technologies and applications that use donated tissue for drug discovery and target validation purposes. Tissue is obtained through partnership with medical intermediaries, hospitals and tissue banks. According to the company, tissue 'surplus to the requirements of patient care' is obtained from hospitals and tissue banks in the UK, northern Europe and the USA, and comes from a wide variety of patients and from all major organ systems, diseased and non-diseased, using living donors and post-mortem examinations. The procedures governing acquisition, use and disposal of human tissue are 'compatible with the advice of several learned organizations'[11] and with 'the spirit of public opinion', according to the firm, although how the latter is determined is not specified.

But Pharmagene is not a tissue bank in the sense that it provides tissue to other parties as it is specifically precluded from supplying tissue and tissue products to third parties by its agreements with suppliers. Although information is anonymized, it has access to clinical information for each donor, with the level of detail depending on the tissue supplier. At a minimum, Pharmagene can provide details on age, sex and either the cause of death or the surgical procedure during which the tissue was obtained. Interestingly, given claims that many researchers are failing to include ethnic differences in the objectives of genomics research, the company does not ask its suppliers to provide ethnic information on the grounds that '[ethnicity] can be very difficult to define and risks breaching patient anonymity' (Pharmagene no date).

Some companies have adopted a business model that involves the collection of samples and personal health information from individuals via the Internet. DNA Sciences (now part of Genaissance) is one such company, with around 18,000 samples already stored in the company's *GeneBank* programme.[12] This type of approach clearly raises additional questions about the meaning of informed consent and patient confidentiality.

A complicating factor in the typology adopted here is that many companies previously labelled as genomics companies are now re-positioning as drug discovery companies (Anon. 2002a). This change reflects the vagaries of capital markets and the increasing unwillingness of pharma companies to invest in as yet unproven concepts. As a result, genomics companies are being forced to move 'downstream' and try to stay afloat by adopting drug discovery business models, with genetic database sales providing short-term revenue only. This relates to a point made by Laage-Hellman (2003: 61) that the relationship between the different actors involved in the collection, storage and exploitation of tissue samples is not static. Changes in technology will influence relationships, as well as the wider environment such as capital markets. Even if the basic framework remains the same, participants may well change their behaviour according to perceived changes in interests and priorities.

Accordingly, many companies are increasingly focusing resources on developing drug targets they have identified themselves, instead of entering into licensing arrangements with pharma companies early in the development process. Typically, companies now consider taking prospective products through phase I, and even into phase II clinical trials before seeking a pharmaceutical partner for large-scale patient trials and marketing. However, this strategy involves higher risks, since longer 'in-house' development means much greater costs. On the other hand, if successful, this approach offers far greater potential rewards than those provided by early licensing. Celera, for example, the company responsible for the private sector sequencing of the human genome, initially specialized in selling information based on tissue samples but has re-positioned itself as a drug development company, and also established a diagnostics arm, Celera Diagnostics, to capitalize on its technology. Oxagen, Incyte and Variagenics (now Nuvelo)[13] have undertaken similar shifts in business strategy, and there are many other examples. None the less, although the emphasis has changed, such companies remain committed to strategies based on clinical genomics, i.e. the generation of data from well-defined human tissue coupled with personal medical and other information, rather than traditional animal-based models of drug discovery.

Commercialization of existing public collections

Another burgeoning arena for commercial exploitation is the use of hospitals as a source of well-defined tissue. Academic and other public repositories, such as pathology collections, have acquired a significant financial value in the post-genomic era, and many institutions are realizing this value through agreements granting access to genomics companies and/or pharmaceutical firms. As Martin and Kaye (1999) note, although such collections usually remain public, the databases built from them are invariably proprietary. Conceptually, this development illustrates the increasing difficulty of defining genetic resources as either 'public' or 'private' as novel arrangements for commercial exploitation are developed, and their physicality becomes less certain and less well-defined (Brown and Rappert 1999).

Several agreements now exist between major hospitals and corporations established specifically for the purpose of supplying biological materials to the pharmaceutical industry and other researchers. Non-profit university hospitals in the US, in particular, have formed a series of partnerships that raise wide legal and ethical issues (Josefson 2000). Similar developments have taken place in the UK, with the Peterborough Hospital NHS Trust Human Research Tissue Bank now a major supplier to the corporate market; [14] and in Sweden, the Karolinska and Huddinge hospitals have entered into similar agreements, as have numerous other hospitals in Europe and Asia.

Early US examples include Harvard University's Beth Israel Deaconess Medical Center and Duke University Medical Center, North Carolina,[15] followed by Maine Medical Center at the University of Vermont, and the University of Chicago, who all signed agreements with Ardais as part of what the company is calling the National Clinical Genomics Initiative.[16] Ardais will bank the tissue provided, collect data, and sell both the data and the tissue to interested parties. Ardais aims to create a massive tissue catalogue, allowing researchers to place Internet orders for tissue samples from patients with the specific diseases they are studying.

The trend for commercializing US hospital collections is encouraged by biomedical societies and universities lobbying the government to relax rules governing the privacy of health records – an essential component for researchers. They argue that existing regulations seriously impair scientists' ability to conduct clinical trials and epidemiological and genetic studies, and have urged the US government to reduce the amount of personal data that must be removed prior to obtaining access to patient records (Kaiser 2001).

Both pharmaceutical and genomics companies are also sponsoring the creation of new collections through funding academic collaborators and agreements with national governments. The best known example of this is deCODE, the Iceland-based company established specifically to exploit data from Iceland's healthcare system in the form of physician records and genealogical records (Pálsson and Rabinow 2001, Laage-Hellman 2003). Public sample collections have also provided the basis for new companies.[17] Oxagen, a UK-based company received important genetic resources from the Wellcome Trust Centre for Human Genetics at the University of Oxford and from other academic sources. In a similar way, exclusive access to the internationally recognized state-funded NIHLBI Framingham Heart Study[18] was granted to Framingham Genomics, although the arrangement subsequently disintegrated over access terms (Anon. 2000a).

The dense web of overlapping deals and agreements around tissue collections and genetic databases, often involving both public and private players, is illustrated by the subsequent activities of Celera Diagnostics. The company has since partnered with the University of California at San Francisco (the medical faculty and university hospital) and Hyseq Pharmaceuticals, to gain access to more than 12,000 DNA samples from cardiovascular patients and related clinical information (Anon. 2002b).

Industry–state collaboration in biobank development

So far we have concentrated on the activities of pharmaceutical and genomics companies. But governments are also taking a major interest in the possibilities afforded by the development and commercialization of genetic databases, and are doing so for a number of reasons. The first of these is to leverage projected health benefits into health delivery systems. Thus the UK Biobank, jointly funded by the UK Department of Health, Medical Research Council (MRC) and the Wellcome Trust, will translate 'knowledge of the sequence of the human genome into real benefits for health and health care' (Rawle 2002). More specifically, introduction of genetics-based treatment regimes is expected to lead to improvements in drug efficacy and a reduction in the incidence of adverse drug reactions. Similarly, the promise of pharmacogenomics and related technologies is also driving government interest in such databases, as the overall effect will hopefully be a reduction in treatment costs and improved patient benefits. Governments also view the commercialization of biobanks and genetic databases in terms of the potential wider benefits to national economies.

The several public collections or biobanks already established, or in the process of being established, provide another, and perhaps the most significant, avenue for commercial exploitation of genetic data in the future. The list of countries or sub-regions with existing or planned large population-based collections includes Iceland, Estonia, Sweden, Norway, Finland, Newfoundland, Tonga, Singapore and the UK plus several others. The next section briefly describes some of these initiatives, although there is insufficient space to analyse them in detail. It is important to note that biobanks have also taken on a regional dimension with the setting up of COGENE, a EU forum for national biobank managers from 24 European countries.[19]

Iceland has received most attention as regards commercialization of human DNA databanks because of an agreement between the government and deCODE, a company formed with US venture capital but based in Iceland. In 1998, deCODE announced it was going to map the genome of the Icelandic people, as part of a larger medical database formed by amalgamating gene mapping with clinical records dating back to 1915 and a genealogical database that seeks to include all living Icelanders (and a substantial proportion of all who have ever lived) to form an integrated genetic database.[20] The Swiss pharma company, Roche, bought the rights to develop and market drugs resulting from genes discovered by deCODE (deCODE 1999). Although there appears to be considerable public support for the project, local doctors and some academic commentators have been highly critical of aspects of the project and some physicians are refusing to co-operate with construction of the database (Enserink 1998, Pálsson and Rabinow 2001, Rose 2001).

In a strikingly similar initiative, the Estonian government signed an agreement with EGeen, a US start-up focusing on drug and diagnostic target discovery and personalized medicine applications. Like in Iceland, the arrangement has popular support but generated considerable opposition in medical circles (Frank 1999). The agreement grants the company exclusive access to the Estonian biobank and health records of Estonian citizens. Formally known as the Estonian Genome Project, the biobank is co-ordinated through a foundation established by the Estonian government and deposition of the first 10,000 DNA samples at a jointly operated sample facility began in September 2002. The plan is to collect samples and medical data from 75 per cent of the population, and leapfrog both the Iceland project and genetic databases planned by larger nations, such as the UK (EGP no date, Anon 2002c, EGeen 2002).

EGeen plans to leverage its access to the Estonian biobank and medical records by collaborating with other biotechnology companies and has announced a number of such collaborations. Related tie-ups with a bioinformatics company, Prediction Sciences (EGeen 2003), and with IBM serve to illustrate the importance of integrating DNA information with clinical and other data and the role of informatics in this integration. In the words of the company's chief executive, the Estonian Genome Project '. . . has a strong wet-lab component, but after a certain period of time it is going to be an IT project' (Uehling 2003).

Sweden has several public collections and attempts have been made to commercialize a number of these biobanks. The most interesting development is the formation of UmanGenomics in 1999 by Umeå University and Västerbotten County Council in the north of Sweden, for the purpose of commercializing an existing population-based biobank. Built up since the mid-1980s, the biobank is owned by the local authority and contains samples and lifestyle information on 87,000 individuals, including 66,000 people who donated blood samples in connection with an ongoing health screening programme (see Hoeyer this volume). The original plan was to identify disease genes and sell this information to pharma companies. Subsequently, the focus has changed to functional genomics and proteomics and, like other companies, to bringing projects 'in-house' because of the lack of interest by pharmaceutical companies. As in the case of Iceland and Estonia, a wider objective of the initiative is to boost economic development and establish a local genomics industry. However, the project has been severely hampered by legal disputes between individual researchers and the university over ownership of the samples – a situation that reflects the rights to intellectual property enjoyed by academic researchers in Sweden (Laage-Hellman 2003).

There are a number of biobank projects underway in Canada. Two of the most publicized are in Quebec and Newfoundland. UK-based Gemini Holdings (since bought by Sequenom) initiated a multi-million pound venture with local doctors in 2000 to identify disease genes in the province's unique gene pool. Interest stems from the fact that Newfoundland's 500,000 citizens are descended from just 25,000 settlers from the British Isles, who colonized the province between the seventeenth and nineteenth centuries. The doctors, who founded their own consortium, Lineage Biomedical, plan to recruit a high proportion of sufferers of diseases common to the Canadian province, such as psoriasis and diabetes. As in Iceland, genealogical data will also be used, but unlike in Iceland, Newfound Genomics will not have access to everyone's medical data (Meek 2000).

In the UK, there are two parallel DNA banking initiatives under development. The largest and most high profile is the UK Biobank (originally known as the UK Population Biomedical Collection), a prospective longitudinal cohort study of 500,000 adults, aged 45–69, from across the UK population (POST 2002). The other initiative is a series of large-scale DNA collections related to specific diseases, in which genetic factors are likely to influence disease risk, natural history or response to treatment. These various collections are archived and distributed through a new MRC DNA banking network (Rawle 2002).

The latter collections are viewed primarily as resources for gene discovery, whereas the purpose of the UK Biobank is to understand the separate and combined effects of genetic, lifestyle and environmental risk factors in disease development. Proponents of the two initiatives argue that the UK's genetically diverse population and universal healthcare system, combined with a strong tradition of epidemiological, biostatistical and genetics research, makes it a particularly suitable place to develop large collections of human DNA linked to health outcomes data (Rawle 2002). This contrasts with arguments advanced in the context of other population databases, such as Iceland, Sweden and Newfoundland, where the benefits of population homogeneity are specifically emphasized.

The UK Biobank differs from the Icelandic and Estonian biobanks in that there is no exclusive access. None the less, many outstanding questions remain as regards its purpose and organization (Barbour 2003), and procedures and corporate access arrangements, although one of the stated aims is to encourage the commercialization of data. The initiative has received strong support from both the UK government and the pharmaceutical industry, although the latter has not made a financial contribution to the venture. This is likely to reflect a deliberate policy decision by the sponsors to keep the initiative 'public' to gain support – a stance that has salience with wider debates about the role of the state, genetics research, healthcare provision and public–private partnerships (Fears and Poste 1999).

As well as the several hundred commercial tissue banks and genetic databases being built by genomics companies in the US, there are several large tissue collections in the public or non-profit sector. As noted already, many of these are academic or hospital based, and often receive major funding from government sources like the NIH. Increasingly, such collections are being scrutinized for commercialization possibilities under the guise of tapping into underused resources for improving public health and/or generating extra income for health delivery systems or universities. Typical of large pathology collections in the US is the Michigan Shared Pathology Informatics Network or M-SPIN, and several others were listed earlier in the chapter. M-SPIN is a human tissue resource providing access to repositories and associated data that is currently examining methods for developing commercial access to its assets (Kort *et al.* 2001). Many accounts of existing collections highlight the provider/researcher interface, an approach that implicitly focuses on academic researchers. But such accounts fail to incorporate the increasing possibility that such research is subsequently commercialized either directly through university 'spin-outs' or other methods by which academic research is transferred to the corporate sector.

As noted under the discussion of genomics companies, large hospitals are increasingly signing agreements for the supply of tissue on a global basis. Large medical practices are themselves also aiming to build genetic repositories. One such example is the Marshfield Clinic in Wisconsin, USA, which plans to collect samples from hundreds of thousands of patients along with medical records and family and environmental data, as part of a personalized medicine project (Marshfield Clinic no date, Kaiser 2002). Collection on this scale is comparable with large government-sponsored biobank schemes and such initiatives are therefore of major significance.

Finally, governments must contend with public opinion towards tissue collection and the several issues that arise around consent and ownership, as part of public policy towards genetic research (Medical Research Council 2001). There is not the space here to discuss this important aspect of biobank formation and tissue collection, other than to note that several guidelines on the use of human biological material have been published in Europe, the US and other countries.[21] Other chapters in this volume discuss these issues in some depth. As a rule, pharmaceutical companies are also active in developing such documents, giving considerable weight to reputation and operating procedures when considering collaborative agreements with genomics companies. The commercialization of DNA is also a legal issue, part of a wider debate around ownership and intellectual property rights, and the definition and 'meaning' of informed consent. As Holm and Bennett (2001) remark, informed consent is 'no longer simply a question of making a single decision; rather it involves expressing one's choices based on a whole range of possibilities'. The right to withdraw samples at any time is widely included in consent procedures, although, in practical terms, if, and how, one can withdraw genetic data once it has been manipulated, made anonymous and no longer traceable, or when withdrawal threatens a research project, remains distinctly unclear. The importance that pharma companies attach to this subject is shown by reports that GlaxoWellcome (now GSK) shunned population genetic databases built by deCODE in Iceland, and a number of others, because of unease about consent procedures (Ince 2000).

Conclusion

Tissue collection and the construction of genetic databases is a rapidly changing field, both in terms of scale of activity and the type and sophistication of the information being extracted. Indeed, one of the few constraining influences is the difficulty of interpreting the huge amounts of genetic data currently being generated from these sources. None the less, the exploitation of existing collections is likely to continue apace, as is the development of larger, more sophisticated, more integrated databases for commercial exploitation.

This chapter has highlighted the difficulty of obtaining an accurate picture of the size and extent of tissue collection and related bioinformatics activities, particularly when located in the corporate sector. Martin has argued that 'we are witnessing the creation of a new type of research system in the domain of human genetics, which also forms the centre of an emerging market for personal and population based genetic information' (Martin 2001: 158), and questions the ability of the governance systems presently in place to meet the challenging questions posed by such databases and the developing market in genetic information. Several years on from these comments, many practical questions around privacy, ownership and consent remain unanswered, and the future exploitation of collections held by hospitals and other public and non-profit institutions, and establishment of national databanks incorporating public health records, can only intensify debate around these issues. As Hilary Rose has pointed out, in most cases, there is no moment when the decision to create a genetic database can be openly debated and decided upon by democratic means (Rose 2001).

The rapid expansion of tissue repositories and genetic databases of all types presents something of a policy dilemma for governments keen to encourage exploitation of new technologies whilst, at the same time, aware of the need to resolve public concerns surrounding genetic research and genetic databases. The challenge for governments is to encourage innovation in a manner that is ethically and socially acceptable. This requires, above all, public trust in the collection and operation of both tissue collections themselves and the genetic information derived from them.

Commercial tissue collection and exploitation, in particular, is characterized by considerable secrecy, and private databases present specific problems as regards claims about ethical standards and data security because they are not open to scrutiny. One approach to help achieve greater public acceptance would be to 'open up' the collection process and encourage greater transparency through the creation of comprehensive national registers of tissue repositories and genetic databases. In the European context, this could perhaps be accomplished through the European Union's COGENE programme (COGENE no date). However, since the public–private distinction is increasingly irrelevant as states promote the commercial exploitation of ostensibly public resources, it would be essential to include the whole range of collections and associated databases (public, public–private and corporate) in any proposed national or regional registration framework. Whilst greater transparency would improve knowledge and understanding of the scale and type of genetic research being undertaken by companies, this in itself would not of course promote public participation in decisions about the formation and use of such collections – this would require increased political and social intervention in their construction and operation, through new regulatory measures such as the introduction of licensing and registration processes.

Notes

1. The NBAC's charter expired in 2001 and was replaced by the President's Council on Bioethics (http://www.bioethics.gov/).
2. The terms pharmacogenomics and pharmacogenetics are the subject of continuing confusion and debate, see Lindpaintner (2002).
3. Although deCODE and others are researching genetic associations using large populations, it is unclear at this time how useful this approach is for drug development. It seems more likely that large biobanks will be used for 'proof of concept' studies once a genetic association has been established through other means.
4. Whereas functional genomics is the study of the biological function of individual genes and the genome, proteomics attempts the more complex task of determining the function of proteins within these entities.
5. Tissue engineering is a new interdisciplinary field that combines the principles of engineering and life sciences toward the development of biological substitutes.
6. Stem cells offer the potential for cell implantation in various therapeutic situations such as neurological diseases, and as a platform technology for drug discovery.
7. The successful operation and maintenance of large biobanks is an immensely complex task, and these skills increasingly reside in companies such as GSK, not in public sector organizations – a development of considerable significance for builders of public biobanks such as UK Biobank.
8. In the case of pharmacogenetics, SNP genotyping of DNA samples is, of course, required as part of the clinical trial itself.
9. For example, the nature of future use of DNA samples is likely to be unknown when collected, whereas the consent given by participants may be narrowly defined.
10. Data in the following sections are drawn from various sources including interviews, corporate websites and industry analysts, such as GenomeWeb

(http://www.genomeweb.com/) and Windhover Reports (http://www.windhover.com/).

11. Institutions cited include the Nuffield Council on Bioethics, UK Medical Research Council and the UK Royal College of Pathologists (Wilkinson and Coleman 2001).

12. DNA Sciences is also active in other areas including storage of DNA samples for pharmaceutical companies.

13. Variagenics merged with Hyseq Pharmaceuticals in 2002 to form a new company, Nuvelo (Nuvelo 2003).

14. Established in 1996, the supply of tissue and related products to the biomedical and pharmaceutical industries by the Tissue Bank was subsequently commercialized through a 'spin-out' company, PCPS, now part of PathLore, a subsidiary of Medical Solutions Ltd (Peterborough Hospital no date, PathLore no date).

15. In exchange the company is building state-of-the-art tissue banks at Beth Israel and Duke and funding staff salaries (Ready 2000).

16. The Ardais agreement is not the first attempt at formalizing large-scale human tissue collection for research from hospital procedures. In 1997 Memorial Sloan-Kettering Cancer Center and Sequana Therapeutics signed a similar agreement, although this was never consummated because Sequana was bought by Sequenom, who squashed the agreement (Marshall 1997).

17. Interestingly, deCODE is often described as such an example. However, as Laage-Hellman (2003) points out, the company is building its own sample collection/genetic database, rather than using an existing biobank. The combining of deCODE's proprietary data with public health records was expected to begin in 2003 (Kaiser 2002).

18. The National Heart, Lung and Blood Institute (NHLBI) forms part of the US government's National Institutes for Health (NIH).

19. COGENE is described officially as 'a strategic accompanying measure aimed at promoting the development of synergies between national genome research programmes related to human health in Europe' (COGENE no date).

20. Geneological records in Iceland go back to 1650, and to the time of settlement in the ninth century for some families. deCODE expects to include information on half of those ever born in Iceland, around 600,000 people (Pálsson and Rabinow 2001).

21. Guidelines include the Universal Declaration on the Human Genome and Human Rights produced by UNESCO; the Council of Europe's Convention on Human Rights and Biomedicine; HUGO Ethics Committee's Statement on DNA Sampling: Control and Access; and the European Society of Human Genetics guidelines on Data Storage and DNA Banking for Biomedical Research (COGENE no date).

References

Anon. (2000). 'Framingham genomics medicine to disband after denial of heart data' (December 29). Online. Available: <http://www.genomeweb.com/> (accessed 15 April 2003).

Anon. (2002a). 'VCs flee genomics shops in Q3; bioinformatics providers hardest hit' (30 September). Online. Available: <http://www.genomeweb.com/> (accessed 1 October 2002).

Anon. (2002b). 'Hyseq, UCSF license heart database to Celera Diagnostics' (9 September). Online. Available: <http://www.genomeweb.com/> (accessed 10 September 2002).

Anon. (2002c). 'Estonian DNA center to begin receiving samples this month' (9 September). Online. Available: <http://www.genomeweb.com/> (accessed 10 September 2002).

Barbour, V. (2003). 'UK Biobank: a project in search of a protocol?' *Lancet* 361: 1734–1738.

Brown, N. and Rappert, B. (2000). 'Emerging bioinformatic networks: contesting the public meaning of private and the private meaning of public', *Prometheus* 18: 437–452.

COGENE (no date). Coordination of Genomes Research Across Europe. Online. Available: <http://forum.europa.eu.int/irc/rtd/cogene/info/data/pub/home.htm> (accessed 15 May 2003).

Coleman, R.A. (2003). 'Of mouse and man – what is the value of the mouse in predicting gene expression in humans?' *Drug Discovery Today* 86: 233–235.

Coleman, R.A. and Clark, K.L. (2003). 'Target validation using human tissue: from gene expression to function', *TARGETS* 22: 58–64.

deCODE (1999). 'deCODE genetics Inc., and F.Hoffmann-La Roche Ltd sign a research collaboration that will focus on the discovery of disease genes to facilitate the development of new therapeutic and diagnostic products'. Press release, 2 February. Online. Available HTTP: <http://www.decode.com/> (accessed 12 April 2003).

EGeen (2002). 'EGeen and Estonian Genome Project Foundation launch sample processing facilities'. Press release, 7 September, EGeen Inc. Redwood City, CA, USA. Online. Available HTTP: <http://www.egeeninc.com/> (accessed 12 April 2003).

EGeen (2003). 'EGeen and Prediction Sciences sign second deal to study pharmacogenetics of depression treatment'. Press release, 13 January, Redwood City, CA, USA and San Diego, CA, USA. Online. Available HTTP: <http://www.egeeninc.com/ (accessed 12 March 2003)

EGP (no date). Estonian Genome Project. Online. Available HTTP: <http://www.geenivaramu.ee/mp3/trykisENG.pdf> (accessed 12 December 2002).

Eiseman, E. and Haga, S.B. (1999). Handbook on Human Tissue Sources: A National Resource of Human Tissue Samples. RAND Corporation for Science and Technology. Online. Available HTTP: <http://www.rand.org/publications/MR/MR9541>.

Enserink, M. (1998). 'Physicians wary of scheme to pool Icelanders' genetic data', *Science* 281: 890–891.

Fears, R. and Poste, G. (1999). 'Building population genetics resources using the UK NHS', *Science* 284: 267–268.

First Genetic Trust (2003). 'First Genetic Trust and Radiant Research announce collaboration to enable pharmacogenomic research'. Press release, 23 January, First Genetic Trust, Deerfield, IL., USA. Online. Available HTTP:

<http://www.firstgenetic.com/Press releases/press 19 Radiant.pdf> (accessed 15 May 2003).

Frank, L. (1999). 'Storm brews over gene bank of Estonian population', *Science* 286: 1262–1263.

Hansson, M.E. and Lewin, M. (eds) (2003). *Biobanks as Resources for Health*, Uppsala: Uppsala University.

Holm, S. and Bennett, R. (2001). 'Genetic research on tissues stored in tissue banks', *isuma – Canadian Journal of Policy Research* 2. Online. Available HTTP: <http://www.isuma.net/v02n03/holm/holm_e.shtml> (accessed 16 October 2002).

House of Lords Science and Technology Select Committee (2001). Human genetic databases: challenges and opportunities, 4th report, 20 March.

Ince, M. (2000). 'Genetic data hits consent setback', *Times Higher Education Supplement*, 18 February.

Jones, J.K. (2001). 'Pharmacogenomics and pharmacoepidemiology', *Pharmacoepidemiology and Drug Safety* 10: 457–461.

Jones, J.K. (2003). 'Tissue collections and the pharma industry'. E-mail (4 March 2003).

Josefson, D. (2000). 'US hospitals to ask patients for right to sell their tissue', *British Medical Journal* 321: 653.

Kaiser, J. (2001). 'Researchers say rules are too restrictive', *Science* 294: 2070–2071.

Kaiser, J. (2002). 'Population databases boom, from Iceland to the U.S.', *Science* 298: 1158–1160.

Kaye, J. and Martin, P. (2000). 'Safeguards for research using large scale DNA collections', *British Medical Journal* 321: 16–19.

Korr, E.J., Campbell, B. and Resau, J.H. (2001). 'A human tissue and data resource: an overview of opportunities, challenges, and development of a provider/ researcher partnership model', *Computer Methods and Programs in Biomedicine* 70: 137–150.

Laage-Hellman, J. (2001). 'The industrial use of biobanks in Sweden: an overview', in M.G. Hansson (ed.) *The Use of Human Biobanks. Ethical, Social, Economical and Legal Aspects. Report I*, Uppsala: Uppsala University.

Laage-Hellman, J. (2003). 'Clinical genomics companies and biobanks', in M.G. Hansson and M. Levin (eds) *Biobanks as Resources for Health*, Uppsala: Uppsala University.

Le Blis, S. (2001). 'Give me your DNA, and I'll tell you who you are . . . or who you'll become – Questions surrounding the use of genetic information in Europe', *isuma – Canadian Journal of Policy Research* 2: 90–101.

Lindpaintner, K. (2002). 'Pharmacogenetics and the future of medical practice', *British Journal of Clinical Pharmacology* 54: 221–230.

Marshall, E. (1997). 'Gene prospecting in remote populations', *Science* 278: 565.

Marshfield Clinic (no date). A new era in medicine. Online. Available HTTP: <http://www.mfldclin.edu/pmrp/> (accessed 15 April 2003).

Martin, P. (2000). 'The Industrial Development of Human Genetic Databases'. Written evidence to House of Lords Select Committee on Science and Technology. Available HTTP: <http://www.publications.parliament.uk/pa/ld199900/ldselect/ldsctech/115/115 we52.htm> (accessed 13 February 2003).

Martin, P. (2001). 'Genetic governance: the risks, oversight and regulation of genetic databases in the UK', *New Genetics and Society* 20: 157–183.

Martin, P. and Kaye, J. (1999). *The Use of Biological Sample Collections and Personal Medical Information in Human Genetics Research*, London: The Wellcome Trust.

Medical Research Council (2001). Human tissue and biological samples for use in research: operational and ethical guidelines. Online. Available HTTP: <http://www.mrc.ac.uk/pdf-tissue_guide_fin.pdf> (accessed 10 February 2003).

Meek, J. (2000). 'Prospectors hunt human gene clues in New World', *The Guardian* London, 15 February.

Melton, L. (2003). 'On the trail of SNPs', *Nature* 422: 917–923.

NBAC (1999). *Research Involving Human Biological Materials: Ethical Issues and Policy Guidance, vol 1: Report and Recommendations of the National Bioethics Advisory Commission*, Rockville, MD.

Nelkin, D. and Andrews, L. (1998). 'Homo economicus: commercialization of body tissue in the age of biotechnology', *Hastings Center Report* Sept–Oct., 30–39.

Nuvelo (2003). 'Hyseq and Varigenics merge to form new company, Nuvelo'. Nuvelo Inc., news release, 2/3/2003. Online. Available HTTP: <http://www.nuvelo.com/> (accessed 15 May 2003).

Pálsson, G. and Rabinow, P. (2001). 'The Icelandic genome debate', *Trends in Biotechnology* 19(5): 166–171.

PathLore (no date). Biomaterials resource. Online. Available HTTP: <http://www.biomaterialsresource.com/DesktopDefault.aspx> (accessed 2 July 2003).

Peterborough Hospital (no date). Peterborough Hospitals NHS Tissue Bank. Online. Available HTTP: <http://www.tissuebank.co.uk/> (accessed 25 March 2003).

Pharmagene (no date). 'Human Tissue and Ethics'. Online. Available HTTP: <http://www.pharmagene.com/> (accessed 15 April 2003).

POST (2002). 'The UK Biobank', Parliamentary Office of Science and Technology *Postnote* Number 180 (July).

Rawle, J.C. (2002). 'UK DNA sample collections for research', paper presented to 3rd International DNA Sampling Conference, 5–8 September, Montreal, Canada.

Ready, T. (2000). 'Teaching hospitals to share tissue with industry', *Nature Medicine* 6: 1072 (accessed 24 February 2003).

Rose, H. (2001). *The Commodification of Bioinformatics: The Icelandic Health Sector Database*. London: The Wellcome Trust.

Stuart, M. (2001). 'Sourcing human tissue: Biorepositories', *Start-Up, Windhovers Review of Emerging Medical Ventures* (July).

Uehling, M.D. (2003). 'Decoding Estonia', *Bio-IT World*. Online. Available HTTP: <http://www.bio-itworld.com/archive/021003/decoding.html> (accessed 5 April 2003).

Wilkinson, J. and Coleman, R.A. (2001). 'The legal and ethical considerations relating to the supply and use of human tissue for biomedical research: a UK perspective', *Journal of Commercial Biotechnology* 8: 140–146.

Wylie, J.E. and Mineau, G.P. (2003). 'Biomedical databases: protecting privacy and promoting research', *Trends in Biotechnology* 21(3): 113–116.

Index